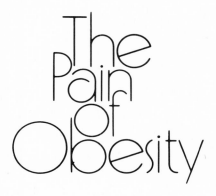

The Pain of Obesity

Albert J. Stunkard, M.D.

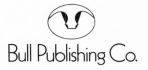

Bull Publishing Co.

Design: Jill Casty

© Copyright 1976
Bull Publishing Co.
P.O. Box 208
Palo Alto, California 94302

ISBN 0-915950-05-7
Library of Congress
Catalog No. 76-3395

contents

To the memory of Harold Wolff

I would like to thank all the overweight people whom I have been privileged to care for, especially for their willingness to shoulder the added burden of our mutual efforts to understand obesity. I thank also the staff and Fellows of the Center for Advanced Study in the Behavioral Sciences. Their company and their help made this writing a time of pleasure and fulfillment.

Introduction

This is a book about troubled people—those troubled by the modern American obsession with overweight and obesity. It tells something about the way they eat, how they feel about themselves and their bodies, and a good bit about how they cope with the preoccupation that dominates their lives—losing weight.

It tells this tale from a special, privileged vantage point, that of the clinical investigator. Part physician, part scientist, the clinical investigator has been given the rare opportunity of caring for patients, and in numbers small enough to permit systematic inquiry into their problems. When I first came to psychiatry there was very little clinical investigation, or research of any kind, and the field was very much the crude, empirical discipline which general medicine had been a hundred years before. We cared for disturbed and unhappy people in a manner handed down by custom. We had no specific treatments for the vast majority of patients who came or were brought to us, and no idea of how to go about devising such treatments. Now, in one professional lifetime, all this has changed. Research flourishes and psychiatry has acquired a scientific base.

Psychoanalysis was just reaching its position of preeminence in American psychiatry when I began my career. It had already become the dominant theoretical system in the field, and for good reason. A new and fundamental understanding of the human condition seemed at hand—not just the relief of symptoms, but the very transformation of human nature itself. At a time when most medical research was leading away from the patient and into the laboratory, psychoanalysis held forth the promise of the most basic kind of clinical investigation into the human condition, in the context of deep and meaningful personal relationships. It had a fascinating intellectual appeal; but more than that, it appealed as a sacred mission of healing, . . . as a major social movement.

But psychoanalysis proved ultimately disillusioning. The generalizations which had stirred such enthusiasm in a generation of psychiatrists did not generate a systematic program of research. And worse, they diverted attention from the real work that had to be done on a lower and much more laborious level, to build a solid structure of knowledge. Only after a considerable time did American psychiatry move in this direction, and begin to develop the scientific base characteristic of other, more productive fields of medicine.

The events in this book reflect my personal experience with this transition, from the high hopes of psychoanalytic training, through a period of unexpected disillusionment, to concern with more prosaic but more tangible problems. Instead of global issues of love and hate, the questions become more modest: do obese people have special ways of eating? How does their social background, and their physical activity, affect their weight? What determines how they feel about their bodies?

For years I pursued this research with little hope of seeing the day when we would move beyond our cumbersome and often ineffectual methods of treating the obese. It seemed for a long time that the most we could look forward to was a gradual increase in understanding; we clung to the belief that one day it could make a difference. Only after several years did the steady progress of the field of behavior modification become apparent. And as its effectiveness increased and its applications spread, behavior modifiers inevitably turned their attention to obesity. A particularly happy union of theory and practice has resulted, and broad-scale management of obesity may now, for the first time, be in sight. But that is getting ahead of the story.

While writing this book I have thought of those who I hope will read it. First, are the large number of overweight and obese people to whom these efforts have as yet brought so little comfort. They should at least know how we have tried. Second, are their friends and relatives. If not already aware, they should understand the pain of obesity. Third, are all those students considering medical research, who may have little idea of the intensely personal experiences behind the limited, tidy perfection of research reports. For some, this account should be encouraging. Others may find the disorder too much to contemplate, and may welcome the early warning.

Finally, I have been writing to everyone whose taxes have supported this work. This book is an accounting to the American people. For a time government support of medical research increased rapidly. Now it is not increasing, and may even be declining. In either case the taxpayers have had very little to say about the matter. Perhaps this account will help them be better informed about the subject, and less vulnerable to political siren-songs about support of medical research. Learning something about how we went about trying to understand obesity may make it easier to assess the press releases about the "wars" that are being declared against various diseases, and the probable effect of massive infusions of money on when the enemy is likely to surrender.

one
Getting Started

I am fifty-three years old, a psychiatrist, and a teacher in a medical school. I am not now, and never have been, obese— nor are any of my close relatives or friends. In fact, until shortly before my chance involvement with obesity, I had no real interest in the subject. What aroused that interest is perhaps worth telling; for although the choice of a field of research is usually not as circuitous as this one turned out to be, I suspect that chance is often more important than logic in such decisions.

The roots of the decision to study obesity went back at least to the outbreak of World War II. Clearly something had gone very wrong in the world, and a good many of my generation felt that it was up to us to put it right. No matter our differences in approach. We believed it could be done. Knavery and incompetence had brought us to this pass; dedication and competence would bring us out of it. But where exactly were we to start?

I am not sure when I began to feel that psychiatry might well provide the solution. In its commitment to help man find peaceful existence with himself, I saw possible implications for the larger world. The kind of intense, scientific study which had proven so fruitful in physics and biology might now be brought to bear directly on the study of the human condition.

With this in mind I began medical school in 1942. Very few entering students in those years planned to become psychiatrists, and fewer still maintained this interest through their medical course. Of those who did, many became psychoanalysts. It wasn't a particularly difficult decision. In fact, most of the recruits to psychiatry in those days were really recruits to psychoanalysis, even if they didn't know it at the time. For it was psychoanalysis, and not traditional American psychiatry, that caught our imagination.

Freud had died only recently and the fruits of his labors were all around us, in art and literature as well as in the field of mental health. From slips of the tongue and pen, to sleep and dreams, from acute war neuroses to chronic schizophrenia, psychoanalysis cast its searchlight, illuminating the most obscure reaches of the human mind. Relentlessly pursuing its task of making conscious hitherto unconscious motives and emotions, it revolutionized our understanding of human behavior. This wide-ranging and iconoclastic theory began to show up in the most improbable places—in the characters of Broadway plays, in the plots of best-selling novels, in the interpretation of primitive tribes. But most important of all was what seemed like an uncanny ability of psychoanalysis to understand the structures of neurotic conflict, and by this understanding to relieve the heartache and pain which would yield to no other measures.

As psychoanalysis evolved over the years, its development was three-fold: a body of observation and theory, a technique of therapy and research, and a professional organization. The initially hostile reception by both the medical and academic worlds forced it to develop in considerable isolation. As a result, Freud came to view psychoanalysis as a field far broader than medicine and encouraged the training of "lay" analysts, often with only tangential relations to the medical profession.

But during the 1940s in America all this began to change. For the first time, in at least some medical schools, psycho-analysis began to receive a hearing and began to pose an alternative to traditional American psychiatry.

Traditional psychiatry, as we medical students came to know it, was a singularly barren and uninviting field. Its ambit was primarily the mental hospital, a region of vague and threatening implications for the public, and one that became no more palatable upon closer contact. The vast majority of patients to whom psychiatrists ministered were demoralized, deteriorated shadows, confined to those vast, remote, human warehouses, our state mental hospitals. The psychiatrists themselves were all too often persons who had not been able to make it in the mainstream of American medicine.

For the mentally ill the situation was appalling, and growing worse. As to the neuroses, the milder emotional dis-orders we saw in our friends and which we admitted in our-selves, traditional psychiatry had nothing to say. By contrast, the hope and understanding promised by psychoanalysis could not have been greater.

It would be difficult to overestimate the impact that the psychoanalytic movement had upon American psychiatry. At one stroke it shattered a chronic pessimism born of years of heartbreak in the state mental hospitals, and offered to the entire field of American psychiatry its enthusiasm and vitality. At a time when war neuroses were demanding the attention of the medical profession, psychoanalysis made available for the first time a theory about neurosis and a rational therapy to treat it.

What I read about the movement and what I heard from the first young converts made a profound impression. The results of actual treatment gave a tangible support to psychoanalytic theory, a far cry from the textbook theorizing about the meaning of Freudian symbols. What the psycho-analyst did for his patient actually made a difference. More often than not, the patient got better—because of something the psychoanalyst had done, and seldom by obvious measures. Often, in fact, their recommendations seemed contrary to common sense. And it was this counter-intuitive quality, apparently so successful, that fascinated us.

In psychoanalysis we saw the promise of effective treatment for the most widespread forms of human suffering, with the implication that even ingrained character traits could be altered. Here was a theory which purported to be capable of not only eliminating the symptoms of human suffering, but of changing human nature itself. Even if psychoanalysis was still a long and painful technique, its aspirations were unprecedented, its potential unlimited. And the science was still young, and we with it.

When I returned from military service in 1948 to begin psychiatric training at Johns Hopkins, the psychoanalytic movement was very much in the ascendancy in American psychiatry; and psychoanalysts seemed to me the wisest and best informed of all the professionals I had met.

Foremost among them was Lewis Hill, the Dean of Baltimore psychoanalysis. Tall, handsome and in the full flush of a vigorous middle age, Dr. Hill was something of a legend among his devoted, and seemingly overawed, followers. At first I discounted much of what they said about his uncanny intuitions, his remarkable ability to communicate with even the most bizarre psychotic, or his capacity to "read the unconscious" of anyone he met. But my first direct contact with Dr. Hill changed my opinion.

At a seminar held for psychiatric residents, I presented a patient to Dr. Hill and experienced the incisive intellect and charm which so understandably moved the young doctors he supervised. As I recounted, I had been called to see the patient, Montague Somers, on an emergency basis shortly after his admission to the hospital. He had already assaulted the attendants, destroyed a good deal of furniture, and been put in a seclusion room. I found him cowering in a corner. Suddenly he let out a blood-curdling shriek and screamed, "You're the devil!"

Dr. Hill smiled to himself, looked up, nodded knowingly, and began: "You're not, you know. He just has you mixed up with his mother." With the assured theatrics of an inveterate performer, he let his statement sink in—and then proceeded. "That's his problem right now. And he doesn't even know whether he's dealing with the bad mother, which is what he thought when he screamed, or with the good mother. I would wager that this young man has already had more than enough experience to know that the bad mother, mother as the punishing destroyer, *is* a devil as far as he is concerned . . . someone who literally put him in this hell of your hospital. But don't worry about all this. In a moment or two you will be God to him."

I gasped as I had heard others do, for Montague Somers' very next utterance had been a, "No, you're God." And he had visibly relaxed, the look of horror on his face replaced by a smile.

Dr. Hill gave every indication of having expected this. He nodded, "It won't be long before he'll be talking about saving the world." And that is exactly what he did begin to talk about!

As the seminar continued, from time to time I returned to an account of what I had learned about Montague Somers' earlier life. Dr. Hill seemed to understand it all even before I had finished. He talked more and more about what the mother must be like, even though I had told him almost nothing about her. "She is an idealist about marriage and love, but you're going to find that she will be very vague about sexual matters. And this young man is going to find that terribly, terribly difficult. Difficult enough that he won't be able to handle it and retain his sanity. . . ." Again Dr. Hill had hit target. Somers' psychiatric break had occurred

in the course of a conflict with his mother over his desire
to marry.

Dr. Hill went on to speculate about the meaning of that
marriage. "He's blown it up into cosmic proportions, because
that's what it is for him. It's either salvation or the end of
the world. There's nothing in between."

Somers' attempt to resolve the conflict was simply to
decide that his mother wanted him to marry, and once he
reached this unfounded conclusion, his progress was very rapid
for those pre-tranquilizer days. Within three weeks he seemed
perfectly well, except for this one misconception.

When I had recounted this much of the story, Dr. Hill
expressed deep reservations about the patient's health: "He
hasn't resolved the conflict by any manner of means. And
this is an absolutely essential task for him. For the major
preoccupation of the schizophrenic is the preservation of his
ideal mother and her ideals. But let's get to the proof of
the pudding. What happened when the patient found out
that his mother did not approve of the marriage?" And by
this question, he anticipated what was to be one of my most
dramatic encounters with a patient.

I had had no success in getting Montague Somers to
consider the possibility that his mother might be opposed to
his marriage. No matter how much I reminded him of what
she had said before his illness, he held steadfastly to his conviction. And, for a time, his mother let him. Then, a month
after he had entered the hospital, she sent him a letter. As
was the custom, I read it before it was taken to the ward.
Dr. Hill had predicted its contents: "I won't say that what
you did with Jane is the only reason you are sick, son," she
wrote. "But I will say that if it were not for Jane and the
things she got you to do with her, you would not be in a
mental hospital today."

The letter seemed sufficiently upsetting to warrant an
appointment with Montague Somers an hour after he was
to receive it. He entered my office in a confused and perplexed
manner. "Let's try to get this straight. Your name is supposed
to be Stunkard and you're supposed to be a doctor. Is that

what I am supposed to believe?" Once again he was out of his mind.

Dr. Hill's response was reassuring, even when his psycho-analytic theories were hard to follow. "This patient is trying to force you to be the good breast, uncluttered by any disturbing attributes. . . ."

With skill and certainty, and a good measure of flattery, he commented repeatedly on the treatment. Finally, two long hours after we had begun the seminar, he paused and then announced dramatically, "This is the finest treatment of a schizophrenic patient that has been done in this area in years."

For a time I basked in this evidence of Dr. Hill's good judgment. And then the doubts began. Such an achievement was, on the face of it, highly unlikely under any circumstances; in that part of the country where Harry Stack Sullivan and Lewis Hill himself worked, it was preposterous. And Lewis Hill knew this perfectly well.

After the first few conferences with the new group of residents, however, some of the magic wore off. Dr. Hill did not seem to work as hard. His brilliant comment might now be replaced by a pained smile, a knowing look, and perhaps an "It figures," as he invited the patient's doctor to pause and share with him some recondite theoretical issue before they returned to a discussion of the patient. Nonetheless he could still leave impressionable young doctors shaking their heads in admiration.

Dr. Hill was most helpful in shoring up morale when things were going badly with patients. He would explain how he had handled a similarly difficult situation; and, when it was all to no avail, when treatment had failed and our patients went to what seemed the end of the world, the state mental hospital, he would relieve our guilt and despair. Never in doubt, smiling indulgently, he would explain why it could never have worked, why treatment had been doomed to failure from the outset. The basis of the problem lay in the comfortably distant past, in devastating experiences of infancy and childhood, which could never be made good. He often explained why treatment had failed, in a favorite statement about these warping influences of childhood, "You can't give what you never had."

Dr. Hill seemed to epitomize those early days of psychoanalysis. His charm and clinical wisdom carried with them a conviction that few could withstand. And with it all he conveyed the conviction that this was just the beginning. Wait until "psychoanalytic research" really got cracking. No matter that the theory seemed to slip and slide according to circumstances, and that at times it seemed more a justification of some intuitive leap than the rational deduction which Dr. Hill maintained it was. No matter either that others could not make the kinds of deductions which he seemed to be making. In time, they would come.

It was heady wine, and there was not one of us who didn't share the hope of comparably brilliant performances. But beyond our dreams of glory lay the conviction that this man and his theory could give us the tools to relieve human suffering. That, after all, was our goal.

Six months after I met Lewis Hill, I entered psychoanalytic training. For nearly three years I participated in the traditional three-part program: personal psychoanalysis, didactic training (course work), and carrying out psychoanalysis under supervision.

It's hard to say exactly when my disenchantment began. Perhaps it had been present, in some form, all along. I remember a conversation I had soon after my earliest contact with psychoanalysis. It had foreshadowed the problem. I had suggested to a friend who was being psychoanalyzed by Dr. Hill that it might be desirable for psychoanalytic candidates to undergo psychological testing before and after their psychoanalysis. This kind of procedure, which could be carried out with little expenditure of time or money, might provide useful standardized information about the changes therapy produced.

The response was one I came to know well: "There really isn't any need for that. I'm quite sure Dr. Hill knew more about me after my first interview than any psychological test could ever tell him. He just doesn't need that kind of crutch."

I tried to argue that systematically collected information was essential to the development of a science. But it hit deaf ears; and as the discussion continued, I slowly came to realize that what I thought of as research in psychoanalysis was interpreted by others as a lack of faith in the field, more particularly in Dr. Hill. The discussion ended in a desultory manner. I had been taught my first lesson in the results of questioning this supposedly iconoclastic and questioning movement.

Gradually I learned a number of unspoken rules, powerful ones despite the subtlety with which they were enforced. Respect for psychoanalysis was the dominant theme. There was no attempt to deny the inconsistencies of psychoanalytic theories, but there was also no effort to validate the sparse data by scientific methods. It was considered both irrelevant and irreverent to concern oneself with such matters. And at the time the stakes had become so high, the goal of becoming a psychoanalyst so overreaching, that we learned the proper limits of criticism and stayed within them.

But as time went by I found myself less and less able to formulate the kind of questions about psychological matters that used to interest me. My interest in psychoanalysis began to fail, and in its place grew a vague sense of discomfort. I kept questioning why psychoanalysts, or more specifically Baltimore psychoanalysts, were not doing research. And even this questioning was all too often dissolved by talk about "psychoanalytic research." Dr. Hill, for instance, offered assurances that modern insights into schizophrenia could not have been achieved without "psychoanalytic research" and the reformulations of psychoanalytic theory it had spurred. His own virtuosity with schizophrenic patients, and the eloquence with which he expounded his insights, could temporarily quell the doubts and enable us to go on, waiting for the day when we could be well enough trained to undertake our own "psychoanalytic research."

One particularly helpful young analyst said that he understood my concern, but that it seemed unnecessarily exaggerated. "We *are* doing research. But you have to understand that psychoanalytic research is a great deal more complicated than other kinds of research. There are just so many more variables to consider." Patiently he explained the difficulty. Measuring one or two variables might seem appealing, and might make you think you were doing something scientific, but this approach could never convey the richness of the data—and it could even be misleading. It was best simply to rely on the psychoanalyst's most dependable tool, his clinical judgment.

My own analyst was less accommodating to these concerns of mine. He kept refocusing our attention on what my concern with research meant, and on the criticism of psychoanalysis that it implied. But my concern remained, and as it appeared less and less legitimate, I began to lose confidence in my motives. My disquiet grew—finally to a point where I sought out the psychoanalyst in the Baltimore area who not only had the greatest experience in research, but also had expressed the deepest interest in it. He, too, emphasized the enormous difficulties in psychoanalytic investigation. But he spoke convincingly of how much more valuable such research was than other forms of psychological inquiry. Not that there was anything wrong with "rat psychology," but why should anyone work with superficial issues when psychoanalysis could open up the enormous scope and complexity of human functioning? If you were worth your salt, he implied, you would do psychoanalytic research even though it was an immeasurably harder job.

"But how?" I asked. "How do you do it?"

He explained patiently that to train for research in psychoanalysis is to travel a long, hard road. First, you have to be thoroughly grounded in psychoanalysis and thoroughly competent in the use of your clinical judgment. And this judgment must have developed through long experience in using the special psychoanalytic situation to help human beings in distress. "No one has the right to do such research," he warned, "until he has listened to hundreds and hundreds of patient-hours, and has immersed himself in the data."

The excitement of my first contacts with psychoanalysis began to fade. Time and again my interest in research was deflected back onto my own psychoanalytic training, and to the necessity of finishing it. In the process I came to take a more and more detached view of ideas which had formerly excited me.

One event late in my psychoanalytic training stands out with particular poignancy, in view of later events: We were assigned the topic of headache in a seminar on psychosomatic medicine. Years before, in medical school, I had heard a lecture on headache which had remained quite clear in my memory. It had been given by a neurologist named Harold Wolff, who was later to play an important part in my life. He had painstakingly described the mechanisms of the different kinds of headache—sinus, eyestrain, muscle tension. The climax of the lecture had been the description of his own major research area, migraine.

Before Wolff it had been generally believed that the pain of migraine headaches, one-sided and throbbing, occurred because the arteries in the head had contracted into painful spasms. But Wolff showed that the pain was produced by the precise opposite, by relaxation of the arterial walls. When he put arteries into spasm by administering various drugs, no pain was produced. When, on the other hand, he distended them by pulling on delicate threads sewn around their circumference, migraine pain was exactly reproduced. Wolff, himself a migraine sufferer, had been his own first experimental subject.

Although Wolff's papers were not assigned reading for the seminar, a paper of Frieda Fromm-Reichmann,[1] one of my psychoanalytic ideals, was. And it posed a problem. For it, too, considered mechanisms of migraine headaches:

. . . Migraine patients primarily want to destroy their partner's intelligence and brilliancy, respectively their brain and head, as the concrete representative of their mental capacity. This mental castration of another person is not allowed and therefore, according to the analytically well known unconscious mechanism, is turned back towards the patient himself; he does to himself by this means what he wanted to do to his partner, thus punishing himself for his forbidden tendencies.

The contrast between this global untestable thinking and the precision of Harold Wolff's, epitomized for me the problems of psychoanalytic theory. But my doubts about psychoanalysis as a theory were nothing compared to my doubts about it as a therapy—for me. After three painful years I had made no progress in dealing with the problems I had brought to treatment. And I was becoming increasingly anxious and unsure of myself.

This was an outcome I had certainly never envisaged, and with perplexity and concern I turned to Dr. Hill. He listened seriously, was considerate of my "peculiar inability to utilize psychoanalysis," and had nothing to suggest. He could only repeat his own guilt-relieving formula for the failure of treatment: "You can't give what you never had." And my skin began to crawl, for this time I was the patient.

In the end I left psychoanalysis, not because of intellectual doubts, but because of therapeutic failure. Profoundly discouraged, I moved to New York and set about rebuilding the confidence that had been so badly shaken. I obtained a position with a research group investigating new drugs for high blood pressure, and spent the next several months working in areas far removed from my major interest. But the interest didn't die. Gradually the idea began to take form that Harold Wolff might be able to help me in my quandary. After a long period of indecision, and with no great hopes for the outcome, I wrote him a short note. Might I meet with him to talk about, as I recall, "issues and opportunities in psychosomatic medicine"?

A reply came promptly from the Director of Dr. Wolff's "Medicine A" clinic, Dr. William Grace. Dr. Grace and I soon had a meeting, during which he spent a great deal of time describing the clinic program and taking a detailed history of the meanderings of my medical career. He seemed to take it for granted that anyone would give his eye teeth to work with Dr. Wolff, and that my tentative note was actually a job application. After examining the program I could understand why he felt that way.

At a time when research in psychosomatic medicine still consisted primarily of interesting anecdotes about patients,

Wolff's large, well-organized research group was studying a number of "psychosomatic diseases" in well-equipped laboratories and in Medicine A—"Admission by appointment." The group working on the psychosomatic aspects of high blood pressure was carrying out measurements considerably more sophisticated than my own, and of potentially much greater significance. Other groups were looking into migraine, peptic ulcer, thyroid disease, and even, as Grace said with obvious delight, "bowel gases." "Nobody else even thinks they're worth looking at," he noted. "And by the time they get around to it, we'll have the answers."

I left impressed with the scope and imagination of the program, and with the high morale of the Fellows I had met there. But I had had a history of being impressed with things, which made me wary. Besides, I wanted to see Harold Wolff. His letter inviting me to visit arrived soon afterwards.

On a bitterly cold February afternoon I found myself walking up Manhattan's upper East Side to the towering white-brick New York Hospital. I entered a pair of small offices piled high with apparatus, books, and papers. Dr. Wolff arrived precisely on time. He was an austere, courtly man, who wore his double-breasted white laboratory coat tightly buttoned, like an old-fashioned cavalry officer's. It set off his slim figure and the severe quality of his peculiar face—thin as a skull, with the skin stretched tightly over it, and heavy red-rimmed eyelids encircling his intense and disconcerting gaze. His greeting had an old-fashioned elegance as he bowed slightly: "Please sit down, Dr. Stunkard."

When he sat down, it was with the brusque manner of a very busy man who has, moments ago, cleared his desk. He listened attentively, frowning, pressing his lips together; to my opening conventionalities he replied not at all. When he spoke, in his clipped precise way, it was to ask about my research. Finally, faltering under his gaze, I asked about psychosomatic medicine, fumbling out a question about issues and opportunities in the field.

"There's no such thing as 'psychosomatic medicine'," he replied peremptorily, and met my bewilderment with a frown.

Was he trying to shock me? He looked deadly serious.

"What do you mean?" I asked.

"Just what I said," he answered with a trace of impatience. "There's no such thing as psychosomatic medicine."

I groped for some kind of sensible response. "Well, what is it that you do?"

"Medicine," he said tersely, with the implication that he did medicine as it should be done.

After what seemed an eternity of aimless floundering, I mentioned the words "stress and disease," and at that point he relaxed a bit. And so did I. We began to talk about what was clearly one of his major preoccupations.

Mostly we talked about emotions and how they were related to "stress and disease." I had spent a great deal of time studying the emotions in the course of my psychoanalytic training. And none of it had prepared me to hear a leader in the field of psychosomatic medicine say that "disease is not caused by emotions, particularly not by unconscious emotions." But what he said in his fretful and impatient manner made sense.

Disease is a result of the stresses we undergo in life. These stresses are of many kinds. Some may arise in our physical environment, like injuries which break bones and chemicals that damage our lungs and skin. Assaults from our biological environment, in the form of parasites, can invade our bodies and weaken, even kill us. But the greatest stress often comes from the personal environment. Man lives his life so much in contact with others, and he is so deeply concerned about their expectations of him, that perhaps his greatest threat is their disapproval and rejection.

Man is vulnerable to stress because he reacts not only to the actual existence of danger, but to the threats and symbols of danger experienced in the past. Consequently, our experiences and our interpretations of them make life far more threatening than if we lived without preconceptions. And that isn't all. Sometimes threats evoke reactions which are more severe and long-lasting than the actual assault itself. The high blood pressure or stomach ulcer which results can be more damaging than the original danger could ever have been.

Disease, therefore, arises not only from stress. Paradoxically, the protective, adaptive patterns of our body, which symbolic threats incite, may become the prime causes.

At this point, Dr. Wolff paused and smiled briefly: "Of course the emotions are important. Conscious or unconscious, they are important—terribly important. But they are part of the adaptive response to stress, not its cause."

When he asked me if I would like to work with him, I simply said "yes." The next question was what would I do. I asked how Fellows decided what to work on. What problems were being studied? Apparently all of the then prominent "psychosomatic diseases" were already being re-searched—migraine, ulcer, colitis, thyroid disease, intestinal disorders.

There was a pause. Frowning, lips pursed, he said, "There's one disease we've been planning to look at, Dr. Stunkard. It might be one for you to take on."

"Which one?" Again his frown, this time deeper and more distressed.

"What's it called? Oh, damn it all, you know the name . . . vascular disorder . . . predominantly middle-aged, Jewish men . . . made worse by smoking . . ."

Puzzled, I suggested, "Buerger's disease?"

"Yes, yes, yes! That's it! That's the one! No one has had a look at it yet from our point of view. Why don't you take it on?"

I left with mixed emotions: delight at the opportunity to work with someone who was doing something important and had far-reaching ideas; intrigued with much of what he had said and at the telegraphic quality of his communications; and finally, vaguely discontented over the prospect of working on a disease evidently so unimportant to Dr. Wolff that he could not even remember its name.

During the ensuing weeks my enthusiasm for Buerger's disease continued to decline. I kept trying, unsuccessfully, to think of ways it could be related to larger issues. Whenever I tried to remember patients I had seen with Buerger's disease, the memories always ended in recollections of fruitless arone had smuggled cigarettes into the ward. I thought for some time about a patient I had come across who had had Buerger's disease of the brain. If I investigated this form of the disease, perhaps I might discover something about brain function and higher nervous system activity. No use. I couldn't arouse the slightest spark of enthusiasm for Buerger's disease.

I continued to ruminate over the roster of "psychosomatic diseases," using the term now with some trepidation, envying the Fellows who had gotten there first, the lucky men who were studying what seemed much more glamorous diseases— migraine, ulcers, and the like. My train of thought led me to thinking about a former classmate, and a good friend. For two years Ted Van Itallie had been working at Harvard with a brilliant young Frenchman named Jean Mayer. In the course of his studies on obesity, Mayer believed, he had discovered the cause of hunger. Furthermore, the discovery was based on a ridiculously simple notion, his "glucostatic" theory.

Mayer had revived an old hypothesis that the control of hunger was to be found in the vicissitudes of blood sugar. Three or four years before researchers had discovered that if you destroyed a very small area in the middle of a rat's brain, the animal would begin to eat uncontrollably, becoming obese. Mayer had postulated that this "satiety" center of the brain, so-called because it stopped hunger, contained cells particularly sensitive to what he called the "available" blood sugar. When the available blood sugar rose to a high enough level, these cells shut off hunger, and eating stopped. When available blood sugar fell so that there was not enough to stimulate these cells, they relaxed their control and hunger returned.

When Van Itallie first told me about his research adventures in Boston, they had sounded exciting. The more I thought about them the better they sounded. When things had slowed down in the blood pressure business, I used to think longingly of working in a field where a powerful theory was organizing the information and reconciling the disparities, where everything was clear-cut and unambiguous.

Now, with the threat of research on Buerger's disease hanging over me, this longing became acute. I found countless reasons why work in obesity was important. If the glucostatic theory really proved out, we could for the first time define a psychological drive in biochemical terms. The hunger drive would no longer be measured only in subjective terms like "acute," and "insatiable," but precisely, in terms of blood sugar.

Such definition would have an enormous impact on psychoanalysis, for psychoanalytic theory uses drives or instincts as fundamental building blocks. But since there was no way of measuring these drives, the theories about them were terribly imprecise and very difficult to use as a basis for treatment. Sexual and aggressive drives had always attracted the most attention among psychoanalysts. But hunger was a perfectly respectable drive, and one that played a particularly important part in psychoanalytic thinking on child development. If hunger could be measured with the kind of precision Mayer claimed, we could tranform drive theory from a qualitative to a quantitative theory, and enormously increase its effectiveness. Freud had often said that developments in biology would one day give psychoanalysis the scientific precision it lacked. Was that day at hand?

The more I thought about these ideas the more exciting they seemed. Here, all at once, was a way of escaping from Buerger's disease, of conquering obesity, and of reformulating psychoanalysis. The next few days were filled with activity. I read the few articles Mayer had written and sent off letters to him and to Van Itallie, telling them of my interest and asking for any material they might have. They replied promptly with a welcome to the field. Mayer also sent the manuscript of a long review article he had just finished, which summarized all of the evidence he had accumulated on the glucostatic theory.

When Dr. Grace asked me to come over to the hospital to sign some forms, I made an appointment with Dr. Wolff. I had decided to ask if I could change the proposed research from Buerger's disease to obesity. I told him about the work which Mayer was doing, how it intrigued me, and that it might make possible some productive research on obesity. Dr. Wolff knew nothing of Mayer's work.

I outlined the theory, exuberantly, detailing its implications and describing how it should be able to distinguish between two possible causes of over-eating by obese people. He listened intently, requested clarification once or twice, and when I asked what he thought of the idea of working in the area, replied without hesitation, "That sounds like a splendid problem, Dr. Stunkard. Why don't you go ahead with it?"

He went on, with no change in manner, to note, "You know, we have no Fellowships available right now."

I didn't understand what he meant and must have looked puzzled.

"We can't pay you for working here."

There was an interminably long pause.

Then he went on to say that one of the nearby hospitals had been asking him if his group "would like to take a look at the problem of glaucoma." He thought that this hospital had some funds. If I worked half-time there, it would leave half-time for work with him. In this seemingly haphazard fashion a critical obstacle had been first disclosed, then removed.

I accepted the job with Dr. Wolff and left his office happier than I had been for a long time.

two

The Glucostatic Theory

Arrangements just seemed to fall into place that spring. My financial problem was solved by working as night executive physician at a local hospital. Not particularly strenuous duty every third night, it provided a room, breakfast and an annual salary of $1,800, quite enough to support the frugal life I was then leading, and with generous time left to read and think. By the morning I arrived at New York Hospital, I was fully immersed in the work that lay ahead.

One small incident played an important part in the process of getting started. In talking with a friend about Dr. Wolff, I expressed some concern about whether I would be able to measure up to his expectations. When I stopped for a moment to gather my thoughts, my friend whimsically threw

out a question: "Are you going over there to measure up to
Harold Wolff's expectations or to learn something about obesity?" As simple a question as this was, its impact was enormous. Suddenly I felt a tremendous release, the lifting of a
terrible burden. Gone were the frustration and helplessness
of the years spent trying to understand psychoanalysis. I would
no longer seek answers in the varying opinions of prestigious
authorities. From now on all that mattered was what I could
learn about obesity. It might be a great deal, it might be
very little. But whatever answers I found depended only upon
my skill in asking the questions—and a modicum of good luck.

Of course I had no way of knowing then how long the
effects of this episode would last nor how far they would reach.
But over the years it became more and more a part of me.
Whether an investigation was rewarded by a straight-forward
answer or ended in confusing, contradictory or trivial results
was less important than the research itself. Whatever happened was just between me and the work. And the work didn't
depend upon others' approval, nor collapse with their criticism. I have no idea how many other research workers have
had this kind of experience nor how frequently. But for those
who have, it must be a major motivating force. It certainly
was and remains a powerful one for me.

My initial week at New York Hospital was a memorable
one. For the first time I was part of a sophisticated research
program, in itself a revelation. Wolff's laboratory occupied
one wing of a beautiful modern building, with individual
laboratories containing the most modern equipment for each
of the Fellows. The supporting staff was bright and capable.
The secretaries knew all about the research and were interested
enough to stay overtime with the Fellows when helpful; and
the technicians were of extraordinarily high caliber. They
began to work with us as soon as we had satisfied a requirement
insisted upon by Dr. Wolff—our personal mastery of every
technique we used. As Dr. Grace explained, "We do all of
our own technical work until it gets to be second nature. Then,
when we're really on top of it, we teach our own technician
until the technician knows it just as well as we do."

The Research Fellows were an impressive group. They were a select assemblage, drawn from the best schools all over the world. None doubted for a moment that he was on his way to the top, and that he was going to change the course of medicine. Except for one other psychiatrist, all had completed their training as internists. But they had found internal medicine lacking in the human qualities each prized so highly, and had come to work with Harold Wolff to set matters straight. As a group they conveyed a striking sense of ability, adventure, and the morale that comes from mutually shared expectations.

These expectations were symbolized for me in a large chart prominently displayed in Dr. Wolff's office. The names of the Research Fellows were listed on the left-hand side, running from top to bottom. Across the top was a long list of the annual meetings of the important medical and scientific societies that had any interest in stress and disease. The chart detailed the status of each Fellow's plans for each meeting: whether he had submitted an abstract of a presentation to the society, whether the abstract had been accepted and he was scheduled to present it, whether he had presented it, and whether the resulting paper had been written, submitted for publication, accepted for publication, and published. In this way Wolff and his Fellows worked with the constant knowledge of the industry and achievements of each.

Expectations seem very important in medicine and in science. Nobel Prize winners are few and far between, and many people live out their scientific careers with little or no contact with one. Yet it has been estimated that two-thirds of the Nobel laureates in medicine and science have worked under Nobel laureates. No doubt this phenomenon can be largely attributed to the appeal that vital, fast-breaking research areas and charismatic teachers have for bright young minds. But it is also due to the expectations of achievement that a great scientist sets for his research workers.

Unfortunately, psychiatry has suffered from low expectations. Twenty years ago the expectations that did exist related mainly to the emotional well-being of the psychiatrists themselves, to ensuring that they were reasonably comfortable with themselves and free of neurotic traits that might impair treatment. These qualities are very helpful in permitting a psychiatrist to devote himself wholeheartedly to the patient he is treating, and only today is the rest of medicine discovering their value. But they have barely advanced psychiatry's contribution to human welfare, and have done nothing to generate desperately needed new knowledge.

The situation has changed to some degree in the past 20 years. But the contrast between what was expected of me when I was at Hopkins, one of the finest psychiatric training centers in the country, and what Harold Wolff expected, was glaring. Even today, very few of the training programs that prepare young physicians for careers in psychiatry expect, and get, the kind of performance Harold Wolff took for granted.

From the first day the contact with the Research Fellows was as stimulating as any I had experienced. Each wanted to know in detail what research I was planning to do, each discussed these plans with deep seriousness, and each, in turn, was fascinated by the glucostatic theory. In the course of these discussions I came to understand more and more about the regulation of food intake, and became increasingly impressed with the logic of Jean Mayer's argument.

The argument, and the thinking behind it, had its origin in the discovery that the brain has areas that control hunger and satiety. This information had been obtained in experiments with rats, by either destroying these brain centers or by stimulating them with an electric current. No one had the slightest idea of what caused them to turn off and on in the normal course of events. But knowing that there were such centers enormously simplified the problem of finding the cause of hunger. Presumably, some change in the environment around the centers signalled them to become active, turning hunger on or off. The number of ways the environment in the middle of the brain could change were limited indeed.

Mayer boldly asserted that blood sugar was the mysterious signal the brain centers heeded. His argument started with the commonsense notion that we stop eating at the end of a meal because we have replenished some missing nutrient. And we become hungry again when the nutrient is once again depleted.

It seemed reasonable to assume that the unknown nutrient was one of the three major foodstuffs—fat, protein or carbohydrate—or a breakdown product of one of them. Of the three, only the body's store of carbohydrates is significantly depleted during the few hours between meals. It seemed clear that the triggering nutrient could not be fat or protein; such a tiny fraction of the total body store is used up that it is very unlikely that any brain center could detect the change.

The body can store only very small amounts of carbohydrate. In fact the liver, which is the principal storage place of readily available carbohydrate, can store no more than the body's daily caloric requirement. Consequently, a large proportion of the body's carbohydrate stores is used up in the few hours between meals. Any center sensitive to the depletion of carbohydrate stores should have no trouble detecting a change of this size, and letting the brain know that more carbohydrate is needed. Furthermore, a similar mechanism could serve the opposite function, stopping the intake of food when carbohydrate stores had been replenished.

But how did a receptor become sensitive to the depletion and replenishment of carbohydrate stores? It could not be by means of the blood sugar level; for hunger occurs in diabetics with very high blood sugar levels. Mayer tackled this problem head on. He explained the diabetic's hunger in the face of high blood sugar levels by the fact that this blood sugar was not "available." The cells in the satiety center of the brain likewise found this blood sugar "unavailable" and acted accordingly, refusing to put the brakes on the drive to eat.

There was another way of looking at these matters, which also supported the glucostatic theory. Under normal circumstances the brain is unique among body tissues in its total dependence upon blood sugar for its nourishment. As a result, the absence of blood sugar for even a few minutes can destroy the brain. And since blood sugar comes primarily from car-

bohydrates, its constant supply is crucial. What better way
to assure the constant availability of this fundamental nutrient
than by making it the biochemical trigger of a fundamental
drive—hunger?

The more I thought about this theory, the better it
sounded. And it led directly into the next question. What
went wrong in obesity?

Two distinct possibilities suggested themselves. First, the
glucostatic mechanism itself might break down. In this case,
the presence of available sugar would be inadequately signaled
to the brain, so that an obese person would continue to feel
hunger and therefore eat, even when adequate amounts of
blood sugar were available. The second possibility was that
the glucostatic mechanism itself might be intact, but for some
reason the obese person might not have enough blood sugar
available. The glucostatic mechanism might be simply sig-
naling this fact to the brain. Exactly this situation, an inadequate supply of available blood sugar, occurred in two disorders: diabetes and the rarer condition of hypoglycemia. And
both conditions were associated with obesity.

Of the two possibilities, the first appeared the easier to
test—was there a breakdown in the glucostatic mechanism in
obesity? This test would involve measuring levels of "available" blood sugar in obese people and seeing how these levels
related to their states of hunger and their periods of eating. If
the mechanism was intact, they should be hungry and eat
when their "available" blood sugar had fallen to low levels,
and they should feel satiated and stop eating when it rose
again. If, on the other hand, the mechanism were defective,
their hunger and eating should show no relationship to the
levels of "available" blood sugar.

We set about testing the first possibility, using a simple
but ingenious method of measuring "available" blood sugar
developed by Mayer and Van Itallie. They had compared
the level of sugar in the blood leaving the arm with the sugar
level of the blood entering the arm. The difference between
these two levels is called the arteriovenous or "AV" difference.
When the AV difference is great, it means that appreciable

sugar has been removed from the blood by the arm; when it is slight, little sugar has been removed. And the amount of sugar removed was what Mayer called the "available" blood sugar.

Using this method, I began a pilot study with the standard subject population—standard that is in Dr. Wolff's laboratory—oneself and one's colleagues. The results of this study were easy to obtain and clear-cut, and they confirmed Mayer and Van Itallie's findings. Immediately after a meal, and for hours later, the AV difference was large; and there was no doubt that satiety was present when the AV differences were large.

As long as they remained large, no one felt hunger. But when they fell, hunger might or might not return—and here the findings became confusing. Sometimes it seemed as if hunger did not return until long after the AV difference had fallen to zero. Deciding when hunger had returned was considerably less of a problem for my colleagues than it was for me, for I was very eager for hunger to return at the precise moment that the AV differences fell to low levels. Focusing on my feelings, it got harder and harder for me to tell exactly when hunger did return. Often it would fluctuate widely, seeming to return for a short while, then go away, then return, perhaps more insistently this time.

It looked as if there might be real trouble ahead when it came to testing obese people in this way. For unlike my disinterested colleagues, obese people would be at least as concerned with the outcome of the study as I was, and they would already have had a terrible time trying to sort out their emotional responses to hunger and eating. Clearly some objective measure of hunger was needed.

Early in this century two legendary American scientists, Walter Cannon and A. J. Carlson, had considered precisely this problem and had come up with an answer. Cannon had proposed that hunger was simply the recognition of contractions the stomach made when it was empty, for which he coined the term "gastric hunger contractions." Carlson on the other hand had been one of the early proponents of the idea that hunger was determined by the level of the blood sugar. In one study he had tried to link these two notions by injecting sugar solutions into dogs. Thirty years before I started my investigation, he had reported that these injections abolished the "gastric hunger contractions." Somehow this work had never been pursued, but it had never been refuted either.

The idea of using stomach contractions as an objective measure of hunger had great appeal for me. This time we would study humans, and use AV differences to find out whether the injections increased the "available" blood sugar. And by injecting the sugar we would get around objections which had been raised to the Mayer-Van Itallie study with respect to the relationship between hunger and blood sugar changes following meals. For when people raise their blood sugar by eating a meal, any one of a number of constituents of the food, including fats and proteins, might actually be relieving their hunger. By contrast, giving the sugar by injection should make crystal clear whether or not it was the sugar that was relieving the hunger.

So, rather than use the original Mayer-Van Itallie technique to test obese people, we modified the experiment in two ways. Instead of producing satiety with a meal, we would do it with sugar injections. And the effects of the injection would be assessed not only by what the subject felt, but more objectively, by what his stomach did. The experiment was getting more complicated, but it was focusing much more specifically and objectively on the glucostatic mechanism.

Measuring stomach contractions was actually quite a simple procedure, although an uncomfortable one. A balloon was attached to a rubber tube which was then swallowed. The balloon was blown up and when the stomach contracted, the pressure of the balloon was transmitted up the tube to a recording device.

In the spirit of the laboratory I prepared tubes and attempted to swallow them, but try as I would, I could not learn to swallow a tube; and each day ended in gagging, weeping misery, head down in the laboratory sink.

Finally with the aid of a local anesthetic I learned how to get a tube down and keep it there. But by this time I had become so disenchanted with the procedure that it was no great trick to persuade myself that I would not be a good subject; a local anesthetic would surely foul up the behavior of my stomach if my nausea did not.

After weeks of agonizing the decision not to be my own experimental subject made it possible to move ahead quite rapidly. Recruiting subjects was easy in those days before the present concern with the ethics of human experimentation and the rights of experimental subjects. Subjects were usually medical students (who were paid a pittance), or patients or research fellows, who were paid nothing. As long as the experiment was not clearly dangerous, the decision to carry it out was essentially a private matter for each investigator.

Looking back, it is remarkable how rarely the ethical issues of clinical research, and of using patients as experimental subjects, were debated or even discussed. There was criticism of psychological studies of patients, but it came from another quarter. Purists who rarely carried out research themselves deplored in the strongest terms all experimental work with patients. They maintained that it was essentially impossible to discover what events meant to the patient, and without such understanding it was simply not possible to interpret the results. Perhaps experiments could teach something about biological mechanisms, but even here there were doubts.

In this climate Harold Wolff had proceeded with single-minded determination to carry out what his critics called his simple-minded studies. His position was clear: a beginning had to be made, so he would make it—and his students along with him. In the course of time we made errors, and discovered them, and in part corrected them. Meanwhile we began to learn something about how to carry out human experiments in stress disorders.

For a time I focused all my efforts on measuring stomach contractions, until the technique was second nature. In the course of this work I developed a fascination for the record itself, particularly as it was traced by the recording pen. When the stomach was quiet, the pen would trace out low, regular undulations in time with the subject's breathing. Then the stomach contractions would start, and peaks would begin to appear every two or three minutes. These peaks would at first be low and uncertain, hardly higher than the respiratory movements. Perhaps they would disappear for a time, then reappear. They would gather height and duration and then move in rhythmic progression for 30, 40, 50 minutes—sometimes an hour, sometimes even longer.

When I could measure stomach contractions without difficulty, I was ready to find out the effect an injection of sugar had upon them. The injection was a simple matter: an intravenous infusion of a sterile salt solution was started, and when the time came, the sugar was injected directly into the intravenous tubing. In this way the subject was not disturbed by having a needle put in his arm at just that critical time when we were looking for the effects of the sugar. The first few tests of this procedure made it clear that the subjects were aware that something was going on in their arm when the sugar injection was given. But very few had any pain or discomfort.

The time had come for my first experiment. There is a certain drama in any research, a drama that may hang on the simple behavior of a recording pen. On this pen rides the hopes behind months of reading and planning, and behind them all the years that lead to those months. After all the issues have been reduced to this one event, and the question is put to nature, the answer is written out by the recording pen. If it has all been planned correctly, the results are stark and unambiguous.

Would the sugar injection stop the contractions or not? I watched. After a time, when the salt infusion was dripping steadily, the contractions began. They built up in intensity, until the pen was tracing its high arching curves. Then came the sugar injection. The recording pen traced out another contraction, and perhaps a minute later, one more. Then, the curve failed to rise. The contractions were over.

I collected blood specimens at 10 minutes, 20 minutes, and 40 minutes after the injection. That night, with bated breath, I analyzed these specimens for their sugar content, and for the all-important AV differences. They were high, just as the theory said they would be. So it went the first time, and the second, and the third time.

Next came the "controls." Sugar injections seemed to be stopping the subjects' contractions, and as the theory predicted, the AV differences were large. But it was possible that it was the discomfort of the injection and the taking of blood, rather than the increase in the AV differences, that were stopping the contractions. We could find out by repeating the experiment with diabetics. Without insulin, diabetics cannot utilize their blood sugar. So their AV difference would be small, despite the sugar infusion. Under these circumstances the injections should not halt the contractions, and the possibility that the injection itself was stopping the contractions could be ruled out.

Once again the drama of the recording pen was enacted. This time if the theory were right the contractions would continue after the injection, and the AV differences would be small. And that was exactly how it went: continued contractions, small AV difference.

That this evidence supported the glucostatic theory was a satisfaction in itself. Actually though, I had only succeeded in supporting the findings of Mayer and Van Itallie, adding some precision by measuring hunger through stomach contractions. The time had come to ask the question: is the glucostatic mechanism working in the obese? By this time I had begun to treat a number of obese patients in the Psychosomatic Clinic. When I asked some of them to serve as experimental subjects, they agreed.

After all the time spent in preparations, the actual experiments took only a few days. And the results were clear: The obese responded in exactly the same way as the non-obese. After the injection, if the AV difference went up, the contractions stopped; if the AV difference did not go up, which happened in some people with both obesity and diabetes, the contractions continued. The experiments showed that the glucostatic mechanism seemed to work for both obese and non-obese people.

What then of the second possible explanation of why
obese people over-eat? Although the glucostatic mechanism
might be intact, was there simply not enough sugar around
to activate it? One way of finding out was to perform sugar
tolerance tests, which measured the rate at which injected
sugar left the blood stream.

One of my very first tests, of a massively obese woman,
showed a strikingly abnormal pattern. In contrast to the 40
or 50 minutes which was usually required for blood sugar
to fall to normal, all of the excess sugar had disappeared from
her blood within 30 minutes of its injection. There was an
added factor: this woman was also depressed. With the greatest
interest I threw myself into her treatment, repeating the tests
every three or four weeks. As she emerged from her depression,
her sugar tolerance returned to normal, and she began to eat
less.

All of these events had occurred during my first six
months in the laboratory. It all seemed too good to be true.

One day in spring, about a year after I first had arranged
to work with him, Dr. Wolff called me into his office and
told me that he was going to be unable to keep a speaking
engagement at one of the local medical societies. "Would you
be willing to go down there in my place and tell them the
obesity story, Dr. Stunkard?" I was more than willing; I was
eager. The "obesity story," indeed. I began to be caught up
in the euphoria.

The glucostatic theory was still in its infancy and largely
unknown to physicians. Not unexpectedly, the lecture was
well-received and the discussion animated and to the point.
It even included comments by Sandor Rado, an old student
of Freud's and one of the nation's leading psychoanalysts. He
spoke at some length on the virtues of this kind of work,
research on mechanisms. He contrasted it favorably with what
he called "traditional psychoanalytic research," which he felt
was preoccupied with theories that were so general that they
could be neither proved nor disproved. It all sounded so
familiar, but not from a leader in psychoanalysis. I left the
meeting walking on air.

The feeling was not to last long. Back in the laboratory, the good luck ran out. I could find no consistent correlations between depression and the rapid disappearance of injected sugar. And then even the basic experiment began to go wrong; AV differences stopped being related to stomach contractions in a regular way. It wasn't that the earlier findings were clearly wrong. That would have been a relief, in a way. The problem was that the new ones were not fully consistent with them.

Neither Mayer nor Wolff seemed troubled by these inconsistencies, and both urged me to publish the results. If a theory enabled an investigator to predict a highly improbable event, and if a few experiments turned out according to this prediction, that was really enough, Mayer maintained. There was no need to continue running experiments indefinitely, simply because some did not turn out as predicted. But I worried, nevertheless. At what point did "some" become "too many"? One day I was discussing this dilemma with Van Itallie, seeking some alternative to endlessly slogging away at the experiments until they reached or clearly did not reach statistical significance.

A major problem was that the sugar injections didn't reliably produce very large AV differences, nothing on the order of the difference caused by meal-eating. Much to my surprise Van Itallie told me of work which he had just begun with a new hormone called "glucagon." He had found that it raised blood sugar levels, which was generally known, but also that it increased AV differences, which was not. In fact the increase in AV differences was striking, far higher than any previously produced by any kind of injection, and comparable to the magnitude of differences produced by eating a meal. If the problem was that the AV differences after sugar injections were not large enough, why not try injecting glucagon?

We plunged into work and in a month of feverish activity settled the matter. Glucagon could stop hunger and stomach contractions reliably and predictably, even in tiny doses, and even with relatively small increases in AV differences. Furthermore, the correspondence between the size of the AV differences and the presence or absence of contractions was dramatic. Finally, obese people responded to the hormone in precisely the same manner as did the non-obese. Here, at last, was Mayer's event, highly improbable on the face of it, which had been predicted by the theory.

This time it took no persuasion to publish the results. We wrote the paper in a week and it appeared in print six weeks later.[2] The paper briefly described the glucostatic theory and the experiments which we had carried out to test it. It stressed the strong relationship between the size of the AV sugar differences and the presence or absence of contractions. And it soberly concluded that this evidence supported the glucostatic theory.

Eventually we did establish reliable evidence of the relationship between sugar injections and hunger. When they produced sufficiently large AV differences, they did stop hunger. But the result was a weak one at best, because the AV differences were usually not large enough, and because a variety of conflicting stimuli could override them. Without the glucagon results the effect would have been unimpressive. Nonetheless, we had made substantial headway towards the understanding of hunger.

Unfortunately, the story did not end there. I was to spend 15 more years trying to track down the intriguing lead suggested by the obese, depressed woman whose blood sugar level fell so rapidly after its injection. What was the relationship between obesity, depression, and blood sugar levels?

The answer proved to be disappointing. I never again found an obese person who showed this rapid removal of sugar from the blood. But for a long time this was not apparent, due to the difficulty in interpreting the results of the test. And before I had found a way of interpreting them I had done an unconscionable amount of work on the problem.

This work resulted, after many years, in what was, I believe, the first mathematical model of a complex biological system, and a long paper on "A Model for the Appraisal of Glucose Metabolism,"[3] replete with imposing equations and closely-reasoned arguments. Analysis revealed that the sugar tolerance tests of obese people did not vary, over a period of time, more than those of non-obese people. The variations were, in fact, so small that they could hardly have played a part in altering the food intake of the obese people.

In short, the results of all those years of work on sugar tolerance were negative. But now I felt none of the devastation which this finding would have inflicted when I first began the work. Instead I felt a vague sense of relief that the study had been completed, and that the obligation which I had assumed had now been discharged.

This long digression taught me a bitter lesson. Dogged persistence does not of itself bring rewards in the scientific enterprise. Admirable as this quality may be, when it is exercised without discrimination, it can divert the investigator from more fruitful activity. What is more, there is a law of diminishing returns in the pursuit of technical improvements. When this pursuit becomes more important than answering the original question, it's time to call a halt and look around. Are there perhaps other research questions which deserve the time and attention now going into technical improvements? If so, it may be time for a change.

And it seemed that it was time for me to change. New research interests gradually supplanted my work with the glucostatic theory. Nevertheless, over the years I have retained a great affection for these ideas, which had helped to launch me on a career in research, and I have followed their progress with the greatest interest. The volume of research, and our understanding of the mechanisms which control food intake, have increased enormously in recent years. In 1955 a symposium on obesity sponsored by the New York Academy of Sciences reviewed much of what was then known about the disorder in 143 pages.[4] Ten years later, another New York Academy symposium required two volumes of over 1,000 pages simply to describe what we had learned about the composition of the body in various states of nutrition.[5] And a recent *Annual Review of Physiology* describes over 200 scientific papers on the control of food intake that were published in just one year.[6]

Where has all of this research brought the glucostatic theory, in the years since I left it? First, it has shown that glucostatic mechanisms exist in all kinds of circumstances, and in all kinds of organisms, from weanling rats to humans. The prescience of Mayer's original ideas has been fully established. But this new work has also established that the control of food intake is a far more complex process than we had ever envisioned. Glucostatic mechanisms play a part in this process; but they cannot account fully for either short-term control, such as the ending of a meal, or for long-term control, such as the stability of body weight over months and years.

Consider short-term control. Blood sugar cannot be the only factor which produces satiety. After meals which contain sugar or starches blood sugar increases and almost certainly plays a role in satiety. But satiety also occurs following meals which contain no carbohydrate, and when there is no increase in available blood sugar. I remember well the countless experimental meals of chopped beef which filled me up completely without having the slightest effect upon my blood sugar level or AV difference.

Even meals which contain carbohydrate, and which are followed by an increase in available blood sugar, pose a problem for the glucostatic theory. For we stop eating these meals before more than a fraction of the carbohydrate is absorbed into the blood, and at a time when blood sugar levels and AV differences are still rising—long before blood sugar can convey a clear message to the brain about how much we have eaten. If we were forced to rely solely upon this kind of information, we would over-eat at every meal. There must be other information upon which to base the decision to stop eating.

Just as the glucostatic theory cannot completely explain satiety at the end of a meal, so it also encounters problems at the other end of the spectrum, in the long-range regulation of food intake. Fifteen percent of the body weight of an average non-obese man consists of body fat, enough to provide for all his caloric needs for nearly a month. This same man consumes a million calories a year. The expenditure of the same number of calories during this time through metabolism and physical activity maintains his stores of body fat, and his weight, relatively unchanged. An error of no more than 10 percent in either food intake or energy output would produce a 30-pound change in body weight in a year. Yet for vast numbers of people body weight does not vary more than two or three pounds a year. And for others, in whom body weight has been raised or lowered by experiment or by the vicissitudes of their lives, there is a prompt return to their previous weight. It is very hard to see how this kind of remarkably precise long-term stability can be achieved by a mechanism with a response time of minutes, or at most hours.

So nearly 25 years after it was first proposed, the glucostatic theory can still account for many aspects of the regulation of body weight. And although it cannot account for all, such power among physiological theories is extremely rare. It hardly matters that the physiology of body weight has turned out to be so complex that we seem no nearer to understanding it than we did in the days when Jean Mayer and his ideas first burst upon the scientific world.

three
Night Eating

Harold Wolff's program did not consist solely of experimental work. It placed at least as much emphasis on the care of patients; in fact, the clinical work frequently took far more time than the experimental work. For Dr. Wolff was convinced that the study of stress and disease was still at a very early stage of development, and that our observations of patients were as likely to advance the field as were the more precise experimental studies carried out in the laboratory.

With balanced regularity, research Fellows typically spent mornings in the laboratory, afternoons in the clinic. Patients were referred from a variety of sources; most were suffering from psychosomatic disorders. A few old-timers had been treated in the clinic since its inception six years before and were passed from Fellow to Fellow. Others were referred to us from elsewhere in the hospital. As soon as it became known that a Fellow was interested in a particular disease, he was called into consultation for patients suffering from it. Since obesity is so widespread, and had not been previously studied at the New York Hospital, I soon found myself in great demand. Within two months of my arrival I was actively treating 25 obese patients. In order to keep some perspective, and to provide a source of controls with whom to compare my obese patients, I began to treat an equal number of people suffering from other psychosomatic disorders.

The focus of the clinical program was the weekly case presentation. In rotation, each Fellow would describe in detail a patient he was treating. In many ways the presentations were similar to those given in psychiatric programs. They covered a great deal of information about the patient's early life, his developmental history, his current life situation, and what its various facets meant to him. We paid particular attention to the onset of the illness and its fluctuations in intensity, in an effort to determine what led to improvement or worsening of the symptoms. Here the similarity to the usual psychiatric conference ended.

In Medicine A the purpose was inquiry, while in most psychiatric presentations it was teaching, and sometimes in-doctrination. The quality of psychiatric conferences so often depended on the charisma of a performer. In Medicine A it was the incisiveness of the investigator that made the dif-ference. The approach of the former was authoritarian and didactic, of the latter democratic and questioning. Where Lewis Hill had informed, Harold Wolff asked.

The expectations for Medicine A's conferences were very high. Frequently a conference stimulated a new research ven-ture or served as a progress report on research already under way. It might also be of clinical findings presented for final criticism prior to publication. In preparation, a Fellow would pore over the notes of his patient for weeks, read anything that might help elucidate a curious finding, formulate and then reformulate—all in an effort to find material worthy of his colleagues' time.

From the beginning I treated patients against this background. Each meeting with a patient served as a challenge to discover something new about him and his problems. This kind of clinical research is hard work, since there is no theory to test and you must be on perpetual lookout for any and all details, without quite knowing their significance. Basically, it's groping in the dark—unlike my experience with the glucostatic theory, which had revealed the relative ease with which testable questions can be formulated from a clear and unambiguous theory. Even a poor theory is better than none, as long as it can be tested. So I began to look for theories about obese people, theories derived from contact with patients. What were the burning questions being asked by clinicians treating obese patients? What hypotheses guided their efforts?

Surprisingly, there were almost no questions. It was as if everything that could be known about obese people was known already. I kept encountering puzzled looks. "What exactly are you looking for anyway?" Certainly there was no great satisfaction with the results of treatment for obesity; everyone agreed that obese patients rarely lost much weight. But psychoanalytic theory explained why: "Obesity is due to fixation of the libido at a very early stage of development. These early oral fixations are the most difficult, but it's a good subject to work on if you can stand the intense orality of the obese."

"Why is it a good subject?" I used to ask, and I would hear, "Because you can learn a lot about very primitive character structures, and a great deal about yourself in the process."

"What sort of things can you learn?"

"Plunge in. Start treating patients and see. Develop your clinical judgment by listening to patients for hundreds and hundreds of hours. Immerse yourself in the data. Peel off the defenses and find out what's underneath." As for specific methods and testable theory, there was very little that anyone could offer.

The full implication of this lack of questioning did not strike me until much later. At the time I just felt perplexed and discouraged—and quite unable to formulate any questions. Even choosing a topic for the weekly case conference was a problem. In the end, however, the search for a topic led to a fascinating find: night eating. But the path was a circuitous one.

My first idea for a topic was a consideration of the bland appearance which overlay the intense suffering of many obese people. Since the stereotype of the jolly fat man was still, even then, widely accepted, I thought that a conference presentation focused upon this suffering—and its apparent denial by the sufferers—might have some merit. Both were well exemplified in Maxine Wilkins.

In the first place, Maxine had never even thought of treatment for her obesity. Yet at age 16 she weighed 220 pounds and was gaining at a rate of nearly ten pounds a month. With her small frame and five-foot figure, this weight made her appear, if not quite grotesque, at least matronly. Her severe black dress and chubby expressionless face, with black hair tightly drawn into a bun at the back of her head, gave her the appearance of a little old woman, from whom all the life had been drained.

Initially she said nothing about her obesity. She had been brought to the hospital by her mother because she had had attacks of excruciating pain in her abdomen. These pains, which had been increasing, had almost ended her schooling and now required morphine. The referring doctor's note, which also did not mention obesity, told the story that had become Maxine's standard reply to questions about her life: "Maxine is always happy, sociable, good in school work, has plenty of dates. Her family relationships are excellent."

In the course of learning about her abdominal pains, I asked Maxine what sort of things made her nervous and how she thought these might be related to her pain. With a sweet smile she told me that the other doctor who had seen her in the hospital had said she was to come to the psychiatric clinic because she was nervous. She said that while it was true that she had been nervous about seeing him, she hardly ever felt nervous at other times and didn't believe the nervousness could have anything to do with her pains. But she quickly added that she was quite willing to accept my advice if I felt there was a connection.

"Do you really think that nervousness could be causing the pain?" she asked. "I mean, it seems to me quite silly, though I suppose you know from studying the various cases, just how nervousness and worry could cause pain. . . ."

With a pretty smile she said that things were going very well in her life. She enjoyed her school work and regretted that her illness was keeping her from attending school and participating in its many fascinating activities. The illness had not, however, interfered with her social life to any great extent. She still went out on frequent dates, visited with her girl friends, and spent very happy hours at home. Home was, in fact, the center of her life, and the evenings with her family were pure delight. She and her sister played cards with their parents; she would listen to the ball game on the radio with her father; and her mother would play the piano and sing. The father had recently bought a recording machine, ". . . and we use it quite a lot for enjoyment." Enjoyment, it developed, was singing: "Just the three of us, Mother, Matilda, and me. And sometimes Daddy chimes in. He sings off key, but he enjoys it. Usually he takes care of the recording machine and lets us sing to our hearts' content." Throwing herself into the account with a radiant smile, Maxine assured me, "I think I have just about the best family in the whole world."

Since she did not admit to any problems, I was somewhat surprised when Maxine readily agreed to psychiatric treatment. I would have been less surprised after my first few months in Medicine A, when I had heard similar presentations by other obese people.

I remember facing the beginning of that treatment with some concern. But assured by my reading that such a patient must certainly have emotional problems, I was prepared to believe that this was the case. But how, I wondered, would

I get her to acknowledge these problems, let alone work on them?

I need not have been concerned. Maxine arrived at our first treatment interview wearing her sweet, reassuring smile. Then she said, "I must start off by confessing that I didn't tell the truth about all the questions you asked me. One of the things you asked me about was girl friends and things like that, and I said that I had them. But I don't. And I never had a date with a boy."

There had been a time, years before, when she had felt that things had been as happy as she had described them to me. She remembered as a little girl singing with her mother and sister, playing cards with her parents, and days when ". . . Mother was carefree and not nervous . . . ," and ". . . Daddy used to take us out to dinner every week . . ." "But things changed after he got the job as a salesman. That was four years ago. He used to take money from his company fund, you know, to pay for food and medicines. It was only for necessities. I mean my father *is* a grand man. And then he would have to return the money at the end of the week. That was always a terrible time. The whole family would be up late on Thursday night trying to decide how much of the money he should bring back."

Once the decision had been made, mother and daughters would scatter on Friday morning, each visiting those neighbors from whom she felt she had the best chance of borrowing. They would return before the father went to work and give him the money, which he would then use to replace what he had appropriated. On Friday evening they would deliberate how to make token repayments to the neighbors in an effort to keep these sources of support open.

"This went on all summer and then into the fall. All of us believed that by Christmas time things would get straightened out, and I kept looking forward to Christmas and praying for it to come. But then Christmas came, and things were just the same. It was dreadful. We just didn't know which way to turn."

Gradually this state of indebtedness became a way of life for the family and the central theme of its long, anxiety-ridden discussions. The small income the father earned from commissions was not enough to support the family's way of life, and the chronic borrowing gradually isolated them from the community. Maxine and her sister became increasingly uneasy in their contacts with neighbors, even contacts not related to borrowing money. Finally, her older sister took what appeared to be the only course that might bring some permanent relief. At the age of 17 she left school to take a job.

Maxine's main reaction to this event was shame, and she found it harder than ever to face the neighbors. "And I also felt just terrible that I wasn't helping the family the way Matilda was. So I used to try to help her by washing and ironing her clothes and doing little things for her."

At first Matilda enjoyed the relief her salary afforded the family, and basked in the increased attention she received and in the favors Maxine did for her. Then the family gradually adjusted to the new and higher income, and the cycle was repeated. The father's income began to fall off. Matilda began to get bitter. "She says it wouldn't be so bad if things were getting better. But they aren't. As long as the money comes in, Daddy won't change. She thought of stopping work so that he would have to earn some money, but. . . ."

As Maxine became progressively isolated from people outside the family, she turned more and more to Matilda, and for a time the two were close. Then Matilda realized that by taking a job she had not really changed the situation, and it began to be clear to her how she was being taken advantage of. She became demanding. The sisters began to argue over the increasing demands Matilda made of Maxine. Maxine began to feel exploited herself and refused her services; Matilda would remind her that she had been forced to leave school to work and support the family, and the least that Maxine could do was to help her in the few small things she asked.

The sisters continued to sleep in the same bed as they
had since childhood, and here they would sometimes discuss
the turmoil in which they were living. One evening they were
discussing their father, soon after he had taken a job as a
traveling salesman, which kept him away from home most
of the time. "Last night Matilda had a premonition that
Daddy had died, and she told me about it while we were
lying in bed. Mother heard her talking and came in and made
her tell about her premonition. It upset Mother just terribly,
and she began to cry and scream, and then we all ended
up crying. It seems like everybody in our family is always
worried about everybody else."

Long before the pains had begun Maxine had been
considering some way out. "I don't deserve to be cared for
the way my parents care for me, when they are so much in
debt and so upset about it. It's impossible to do well in school
feeling the way I do, and the girls seem so young and silly.
I might as well leave—or commit suicide. I think of suicide
a lot, particularly when I'm in bed at night, but I've never
had the courage to go through with it."

What was the relationship of this turmoil to her weight?
Maxine wasn't sure. She thought that her weight had been
about normal before the troubles began, when she was about
12 years old. She did remember having been a "chubby" child.
But the years that had been so filled with distress were blank
as far as her weight was concerned. "I was really surprised
when the doctor weighed me and I found out that I weighed
220 pounds. I didn't know how that had happened. I knew
I was eating more than usual, but I would just say 'What's
the use?' and go on. There's so much I'm not aware of, I
don't know whether I realized that I was becoming heavy
or not." It was not even clear she knew her over-eating was
causing her overweight.

As I reviewed these notes, they clearly demonstrated the
pain behind the bland appearance. It was the same pain I
was seeing in so many obese people. A presentation focused
on this discrepancy might have some merit in debunking the
stereotype of the jolly fat man; but by this time it seemed

increasingly important to focus on more specific topics. I was beginning to see other obese patients whose relations with their parents had much in common with those of Maxine. So I examined the notes on these relationships to try to understand them as fully as possible.

One central theme was the emphasis on family "closeness." In Maxine's family both daughters had been discouraged from having outside social interests, even before the financial troubles had made this inevitable. Within this confined family system the influence of each of the parents was enhanced.

It became unmistakably clear that one of Maxine's major ways of coping was to identify with her mother. And her mother was a huge woman, 275 pounds, with the same bland manner as her daughter. She denied any difficulties at home, dismissed her own obesity with only a hint of martyred self-sufficiency, as "just glands," and corroborated Maxine's initial story that the girl had a happy and sociable life. She even accepted therapy when it was offered to her, and attended faithfully for two or three months. She began treatment by shedding her mask, much as Maxine had done. She acknowledged what she saw as insuperable family problems. And she wept. According to the psychiatrist who saw her, that was about all she did during her treatment: She would begin to cry as soon as she entered the office, and cried almost uninterruptedly until the time was up. Nothing that her psychiatrist did would interrupt the flow of tears. Eventually they agreed to terminate the treatment, despairing of ever being able to get beyond her tears.

Maxine's intense self-consciousness seemed a direct reflection of her mother's. "Mother has always said that a heavy person should keep in the background and not do anything that would call attention to herself. She doesn't dance at parties, or do anything like that; she feels she would be making a fool of herself. And I guess I feel the same way. I just feel ridiculous all the time."

Only when Maxine's treatment began to make her more independent of her family, and less likely to be caught up in the recurrent family turmoil, was her mother able to mobilize herself. Apparently desperate because of the threat to the integrity of the family, both mother and father began to lash out at the treatment. Their message was the same: Maxine's motives for coming to the hospital were not therapeutic but sexual.

"Mother has been teasing me again about coming in to the hospital. She said that I was just coming in because I liked you, and that it's disgusting. She said that she couldn't let me waste the family's money on carfare for this sort of silliness. She said, 'If you and Dr. Stunkard are so close, let him come out here to see you.' "

As Maxine persisted in treatment, and her independence grew, her mother's attacks mounted. "Now she says that the reason I'm coming in is either because I'm a hopeless case or because I'm after your body, and she wants to know which one it is. She just keeps telling me how disgusting it is. I am afraid that she won't let me keep coming in and I don't know what to do about it."

Mrs. Wilkins was so ineffectual that even her desperation about the loss of Maxine could not rouse her to terminate treatment. Not so with Mr. Wilkins. Maxine's father was a man with an extraordinary ability to get what he wanted, and he managed to live the life of a pampered princeling even in these improbable circumstances. A large handsome man, his overweight skillfully disguised by excellent tailoring, he extracted from his environment a remarkable series of indulgences. Only late in the treatment did an embarrassed Maxine reveal that "Daddy has breakfast in bed every morning when he's home." She accepted this as a perfectly reasonable way of life, and was upset only because ". . . he never shows any appreciation to Mother for going to this trouble. He just seems to take it for granted. It's nice to have a happy-go-lucky attitude and to enjoy things, but sometimes I *do* wish that Daddy would be more serious. Sometimes it even irritates me the way he goes on. Oh, I know I shouldn't say things like that."

Usually Maxine met her father's demands, just as her mother and sister did. Why did these three women continue to support and pamper this man? One possibility was that the drabness of the family's life was somehow made to seem worthwhile when they provided enjoyment for Daddy, because Daddy seemed to be the only member of the family who could really enjoy himself. And Maxine was more than a little attracted to this winsome rogue. In this inhibited, confused, and demoralized family, the father's lack of inhibitions, his ability to seek gratification for himself regardless of the consequences to others, exercised a kind of magic. Whatever he said or did, he seemed more than life-size.

What he said to Maxine often confirmed her mother's querulous judgments: "He was just terrible last night. My own father said that if he were a boy he wouldn't give me a second look. He said I was getting fatter by the minute, and the treatment wasn't helping me at all. He said that I would be a good candidate for a circus pretty soon."

Mr. Wilkins had other motives for not wanting family matters discussed outside the house. It was difficult to reconstruct just what had happened from the anguished reports of a frightened teenager, and much of what Maxine reported may have been fantasy. What she told me of were some unusual steps her father was taking in relation to her sexual inhibitions. On four or five occasions during one confusing month he brought home a young friend from work, plied Maxine with drink, told dirty jokes and indicated that he would look favorably upon her accommodating his friend. She froze and resisted.

I learned about most of these events only much later, for in contrast to his wife's ineffectual remonstrances, Mr. Wilkins had moved decisively to terminate Maxine's treatment. She came in one evening profoundly discouraged. "Daddy has been just terrible. He says that this isn't psychiatric treatment, it's lovemaking. And the doctor ought to come to my house, so he would have to pay the carfare. Mother just keeps sitting there saying that it's all so disgusting."

Two days later the letter came from Maxine, breaking off treatment: "Regardless of anything I may have said about my parents, I love them deeply and cannot continue to bring them pain. I feel that my parents have always tried to act in my best interests, regardless of how it might seem to me at the time. I deeply regret that this decision has become necessary. It may be due to my weakness, and if this is so, I deeply regret it."

That was to be the last I heard of Maxine, but her story reflected a pattern with which I was already growing familiar. Within the first few months at the New York Hospital I had seen several family constellations similar to that of the Wilkins family. Time and again I had been struck by how many young obese women reflected the dominant themes in Maxine's life.

To a remarkable degree obesity runs in families: 90 percent of the children of two obese parents are themselves obese, compared to only 10 percent of the children of non-obese parents. On the fertile soil of obesity there grew, with surprising regularity, the same discouraged identification with a demoralized, obese mother—and the same hopelessness. Often, far more often than I would have expected, I discovered also the intense, fantasy-ridden longing for salvation through the love of a handsome hero.

As fascinating as these parallels were, however, they did not seem suitable topics for a conference. I continued search-ing, and at one point thought of discussing obesity as a family problem. But neither this nor other ideas satisfied me. Then, in the midst of my quandary, the answer came suddenly.

For some time a group of us had gathered each week to listen to recordings of our interviews with patients. I had recorded one interview with Maxine, during the troubled time shortly before she had broken off treatment. Concerned by what had happened, I asked my colleagues to discuss the problem.

The meeting began with a description of Maxine's back-ground and the problem in treatment. Then we began to listen to the recording. Suddenly one of our group became upset, a young woman psychiatrist who was obese. Gasping for air, she rose from the circle and began to stagger out of the room. Puzzled, I followed her. She had reached the door and was opening it by the time I could talk with her. Her face mirrored anguish bordering on panic. Only reluctantly was she persuaded to come back to the room.

Finally, with the recorder turned off, she tried to explain to a baffled, solicitous group what had happened, what had precipitated her attack of acute anxiety. "It wasn't anything about the father. That was nothing. It was how that girl talked about the way she eats: Nothing for breakfast. She is never hungry at all in the morning. Then what it's like at night, how she can't seem to stop eating. Supper doesn't satisfy her, and she just goes on and on. She even gets up out of bed to eat . . . That's how I eat, and I never heard about it from anybody else in my whole life!"

For some time we discussed with the obese psychiatrist her reaction to the recording, and then moved on to the problem of the interrupted treatment. But the incident of the anxiety attack stuck in my mind. I could never forget that shock of recognition—the sudden realization that an eating pattern could be so much more meaningful to another obese woman than the lurid events we had been discussing. Here it seemed might be a topic of real interest for the Medicine A conference.

Did other obese patients show this pattern? I was quite sure that they did. But the careful dietary histories I had taken from each of my patients had focused on the amount and the kinds of foods eaten, and they had not paid any special attention to the pattern of eating. Nevertheless I seemed to remember patients telling me of skipping breakfasts and of eating at night. It was easy enough to find out. As each of my patients returned to the clinic, I asked them about their eating patterns. As so rarely happens, the questions were on target.

With a rush of recognition, the first patient I asked told me that she never ate breakfast, never snacked in the morning, and had little or no appetite for lunch. Then as the day wore on, particularly after supper, she ate more and more heavily.

Occasionally she would even get up out of bed, go to the refrigerator and fix herself a sandwich. On such evenings her agitation and turmoil were unbearable.

The next obese patient also reported a lack of appetite for breakfast, eating heavily in the evening, and being upset at that time. With mounting enthusiasm, I posed the questions to each of the obese patients I was treating. I learned that if they ate in this pattern, they were well aware of it and only too ready to describe it. If they didn't eat in this manner, they were also quite well aware of the fact. There was nothing ambiguous; either the phenomenon was there or it was not.

The next steps were quite simple. If the phenomenon could be easily identified, how common was it? I made a list of my patients, and after questioning them wrote down which aspects of the phenomenon (which became known as "the night-eating pattern") were present. It was soon apparent that most of them exhibited three common characteristics: lack of appetite in the morning, over-eating in the evening, and combined agitation and insomnia. These held true for none of the non-obese patients.

As I explored the night-eating pattern further, however, a complication developed. Some patients said that although they were eating this way at present, they had not always done so. Others reported that they had eaten this way in the past, but were not doing so now. What made the difference? About this time one of my patients had an experience that helped to answer the question.

Maureen Reilly was a 29-year-old housewife. She had been referred to Medicine A for treatment of obesity, which was causing frequent and severe attacks of inflammation in the veins of her legs. The eighth of ten living children, she remembered her mother with great bitterness for having, she was convinced, exploited her. Whatever the truth of these complaints, her childhood had been a time of hardship and deprivation. The father's sporadic employment never permitted the family more than a marginal existence.

At age 18 Mrs. Reilly had married the neighborhood alcoholic in an effort to escape her home environment. It was a jump from the frying pan into the fire, and she soon bitterly regretted it. But children followed, and she found herself enmeshed in inescapable obligations. Within eight years of her marriage she had added 100 pounds to her sturdy 5'6" frame, reaching a weight of 280. Her weight had stayed at this level for three years when she came to the clinic.

Mrs. Reilly's manner was pleasant and friendly, but her communication had an oddly impersonal quality. She was usually late for appointments, and her attendance was irregular.

When she came to the clinic she displayed a clear-cut night-eating pattern. She regularly awoke in the morning with no appetite and ate no breakfast and little lunch. Supper, in the early evening, was large, but only temporarily satisfying. During the rest of the evening, often until early morning, she nibbled at various foods distinguished mainly by their sweetness. She was unclear about why she ate at these times, but she thought it might be due to anxiety.

Her anxiety was most severe when she was alone, when she would worry about someone breaking into the house and harming her. The measures she took provided only partial relief: besides eating, she would have company in the house, and when alone, she would keep the radio and lights on. Sometimes the presence of her husband reassured her, but as often she would quarrel with him and then feel even more upset. She would stay up eating until midnight at least, and often until two or three in the morning. Throughout my early contact with her, she rarely slept more than four hours a night.

Just at the point when I was beginning my systematic inquiry into the night-eating pattern, Mrs. Reilly developed a recurrence of her phlebitis, which made it necessary for her to enter the hospital. Not surprisingly she greeted this development with relief and gladly laid down her domestic responsibilities.

Within a day her eating pattern changed strikingly. The morning after she entered the hospital, she awoke with a desire to eat breakfast, for the first time in months. She went on to eat an average-sized lunch and a small supper, and had no desire to eat during the evening or night. This absence of night eating was all the more remarkable in that the pain in her legs kept her awake much of the night during her first week in the hospital. Thereafter she slept well, never complained of hunger, adhered with no difficulty to an 800-Calorie diet, and lost 28 pounds in a month.

This marked change in her eating pattern was paralleled by a great decrease in anxiety. In fact Mrs. Reilly seemed more at ease than I had ever seen her. She attributed part of the change in her eating pattern, and in her comfort, to the presence of her roommate. "She keeps me feeling good in the evenings by talking to me. Then I don't feel like eating."

Mrs. Reilly wanted very much to remain in the hospital, and she used every conceivable stratagem to delay her discharge. Finally, reluctantly, she returned home. Within 24 hours the night-eating pattern had returned. The morning after her arrival home she awoke with no appetite, did not begin to eat until evening, and then stayed up until three the next morning, nibbling. Her husband, who had stopped drinking while she was in the hospital, began again as soon as she returned home. The relations between them, which had improved during her hospitalization, deteriorated rapidly. During her first month home Mrs. Reilly regained ten pounds.

Was this then the reason for the apparent capriciousness with which the night-eating pattern came and went? Was it a response to life stress? And did it disappear, along with the anxiety and agitation, when the stress was relieved? For Mrs. Reilly the answer seemed to be "yes." When I asked my other patients, they agreed.

The more I learned about the night-eating pattern, the more I looked forward to discussing it at Dr. Wolff's conference, and finally the time arrived. I began by describing the tendency of some obese people to eat heavily during the evening, and how they often felt upset and agitated at these times. I mentioned the curious paradox that people, supposedly driven by increased hunger, reported that their appetite in the morning was impaired or absent. I speculated that the pattern might be a response to stress peculiar to obese people, and in all probability, to only some of these. I ended by illustrating these points with the cases of Maxine Wilkins and Maureen Reilly.

The moment I finished, the questions began. "What," Dr. Wolff asked, "is the biological significance of this phenomenon?" I had no idea. I had been so busy getting straight on the facts that such a question had never occurred to me. It was probably premature to ask it at this stage of the game, but the fact that Dr. Wolff had asked it meant a great deal to me. It indicated that he thought that this night-eating business was a real phenomenon, not just something I had dreamed up.

The other questions were individually less ambitious, but taken together they spelled out a whole program of research. "How common is the pattern?" "How often does it occur in obese patients in Medicine A?" "How often in obese people in general?" "Does it really never occur in people of normal weight?" "Is it more common among the very obese? Or those with emotional problems? Or men? Or women? Or the old? Or the young?" Finally, and prophetically, "Does it have any implications, good or bad, for treatment?"

I returned to the inquiry immeasurably stimulated. Once I felt confident that there truly was a night-eating pattern, the subsequent exploration followed almost automatically. It was largely a process of setting down the findings in a way that made it easy to discover relationships between them. In those days before computers a "master sheet" did yeoman's service. On the left-hand margin of a large piece of paper I listed the name of each obese patient. Across the top I listed any issues that might conceivably be related to the night-eating pattern. This graphic display made it easy to see at a glance whether the night-eating pattern was related to any other characteristics of the patients. By and large there was no relationship. The night-eating pattern occurred in young and old, short and tall, slightly overweight and severely obese. Over-all it occurred in 20 of the 25 obese patients, or 80 percent.

About this time I began a study described in more detail in the next chapter, of 100 unselected obese people in the Nutrition Clinic. This study made it possible to answer the

question: how common was the night-eating pattern among
obese people in general, as opposed to Medicine A's patients
pre-selected for stress-related disorders? In contrast to the 80
percent of Medicine A patients, only 10 percent of the more
general sample showed the pattern.

I continued to explore the characteristics of Medicine
A patients. Was the night-eating pattern more common among
men or women? Only two of the twenty-five were men. Neither
man showed the pattern, and most of the women did. But
the numbers were too small to answer the question con-
clusively.

Then, suddenly, one finding stood out in bold relief: Five
of the twenty-five patients did *not* show the night-eating pattern—and four of these five were losing weight. In fact they
had lost a great deal of weight, from 45 to as much as 105
pounds. Of the twenty patients with the night-eating pattern,
only two had lost as much. Despite my intense involvement
with the treatment of these patients, I had been completely
unaware of this association until I saw it on the master sheet.

Five patients with the night-eating pattern had lost lesser
amounts of weight, from 20 to 30 pounds, and had then
discontinued their diets. But these attempts at dieting were
noteworthy. It looked as if the weight loss of four of them
had occurred during a temporary remission in their night-eating pattern.

What about past efforts to lose weight? The column
labeled "Previous Weight Losses" showed a picture very like
that of the present weight losses. Again, four of the five patients
without the night-eating pattern had been able to lose weight
in the past. And only 11 of the 20 with the night-eating pattern
had been successful.

Although my inquiry into night eating had arisen out
of curiosity and the search for a conference subject, one practical consequence was already apparent. When the outcome
of treatment is as uncertain as it is in obesity, it is useful
to be able to predict which patients are likely to succeed.
The night-eating pattern presaged failure, not success. But
inasmuch as it indicated the outcome of treatment, it provided

a useful diagnosis. It could spare obese people with a poor outlook for weight reduction another unhappy attempt at dieting, and another experience with failure. And limited treatment resources could be allocated to those most apt to benefit from them.

I continued to examine the master sheet, adding other items that might conceivably be related to the night-eating pattern. The difficulty in losing weight fascinated me. It was not something that began when these patients came to Medicine A. Only 11 of the 20 night-eaters had successfully reduced at any time in their lives. These weight losses had been unusual events. How had the patients been able to accomplish them? What had happened when they did? I began to ask them more about these successful diets.

As I pursued this question, an engrossing story emerged. The night-eaters had been able to lose weight only at extraordinary cost. For eight of these eleven patients, weight loss had been accompanied by disabling emotional illness! Reconstructing the character of these illnesses long after the event was difficult. They seemed to run the gamut of symptoms: depression, fatigue, anxiety, feelings of futility. Furthermore, the illnesses seemed to arise in a great variety of circumstances. Clearly it was going to take time to understand these disorders.

I had already begun to write the paper on the night-eating pattern when events brought home in a brutal manner the emotional complications of dieting. One of my few patients who seemed to be doing really well was a 49-year-old woman. She had come to Medicine A with a variety of complaints: migraine headaches, generalized muscular aching, a nervous disorder of the skin that she had had for 20 years, and depression. The fact that she was obese and showed the night-eating pattern seemed almost incidental.

The center of a large Italian family, Mrs. Rosselini had years ago settled into a grim depressed mood, martyred and long-suffering. Having decided to devote her life to her eight children, she gained a measure of satisfaction by serving them through the never-ending housework she knew so well. Before she had passed the child-bearing age her older children were already bringing their babies for her to look after. As the years went by she became even busier, and even more depressed.

I began seeing Mrs. Rosselini for weekly 45-minute psychotherapy sessions. At first all I heard were tired, repetitious accounts of her symptoms and of her past experiences, most of them unfavorable, with doctors. By the end of a month, however, she began to speak of her home. Soon she was regaling me with dramatic accounts of how she was mistreated and how she suffered. Gradually she began to see that she had collaborated in setting up her unenviable home life, and began to explore the possibility of changing it.

For a beginning, Mrs. Rosselini began to refuse her children when their demands struck her as excessive. And she even asked them for help when her housework became too demanding. She began to talk about the possibility of getting out of the house, and her old dream of working in a hospital as a nurse's aide was reborn. I was delighted by these developments, and encouraged her to undertake activities that might foster her growing independence of her family. Then her family began to react against their mother's newfound freedom. I met with her eldest son and persuaded him to support her against this opposition.

Two months into her treatment, I spoke to Mrs. Rosselini about the possible benefits of weight reduction. I said I hoped she would try to lose some weight. She was enthusiastic about the idea and began to diet at once. In the next two months her weight fell from 183 to 170 pounds. And her other symptoms just seemed to melt away. Her depression lifted. Her muscles stopped aching. Her skin stopped itching. Her headaches went away.

Only gradually did it begin to dawn on me that Mrs. Rosselini was becoming unusually active. So few of my patients were doing well that I didn't want to question what seemed like a therapeutic triumph. But finally I could no longer ignore her accounts of exuberant and seemingly tireless activities, her decreasing need for sleep, her increasingly seductive dress. I began to be concerned that she was becoming manic. Then the bottom dropped out.

One day about four months after we had begun treatment, Mrs. Rosselini arrived at the clinic in a tight-fitting, low-cut, black dress. Her gray hair, newly blued, was piled in cascades upon her head; she was wearing a pearl necklace, a pearl bracelet, pearl earrings. Breathlessly she told me of further weight loss since her last visit and beamed at my approval. She asked if she had lost enough weight to satisfy me. Puzzled and uneasy, I asked her what she meant.

She began a tortured account of what lay behind the dramatic changes in her life. At our very first interview she had formed the notion that I must be in love with her, and everything that happened afterwards confirmed this belief. Why else, she argued, would I have disapproved of the mistreatment she suffered at the hands of her family? Why else would I have met with her eldest son to encourage the family to lighten her load? Why else would I have wanted her to be slimmer and more attractive? She had done what I had asked; she had lost weight. Now it was up to me. She was ready to go away with me. She was ready to marry me if I wished. To my question about her family, she said that she had no more worries about what her family would think. She was free of her family. She had suffered for them; now it was time for her to live for herself.

I fumbled out some poor response, mortified by my blindness.

Mrs. Rosselini's disillusionment was prompt and profound. She could not believe that she had so misread my intentions. She burst into tears. She asked me again to take her away. Then she left the office.

Mrs. Rosselini did not keep her next appointment. She did not return to the clinic until her family brought her, three weeks later. By then she was severely depressed. She told me that after her last visit she had been very frightened, and had cried almost constantly. She said she was sleeping poorly and had nightmares in which strange men attacked and robbed her. Her speech and actions were slow; she professed no interest in anything. She had given up any effort to take care of her house.

Unlike most persons suffering from depression, Mrs. Rosselini did not express any ideas of guilt or self-condemnation. If anyone were to blame, it was I. Her reaction, she maintained, was a perfectly normal one. How else was a woman to act when she was abandoned by the man she loved? But even now, she said, there was still time for me to rescue her.

Mrs. Rosselini continued to come to the clinic for a few more months, unhappy, depressed, accusing, asking if I had changed my mind. Then her family took her to another doctor. From then on I learned about her only through the courtesy of several of the doctors whom she consulted. Apparently she remained depressed for more than a year, during which time she went through an extraordinary assortment of medical treatments, none of which provided much relief. Some were psychiatric—psychotherapy, electroshock, three months in a psychiatric hospital. Others were surgical. During one six-month period she underwent three major operations, undertaken in large part at her insistence, for conditions such as hernia, that were not causing her any discomfort. In addition she was treated by internists and general practitioners.

Eventually Mrs. Rosselini's sufferings restored the sympathy and concern of her family. Its members began to treat her once again with the consideration they had abandoned when she had tried to assert her independence. By the time her more severe depressive symptoms had abated, she had already returned to her drab, colorless existence. She remained mildly depressed; her muscles began to ache again, her skin resumed its itching, her migraine returned. Her weight rose once again to over 180 pounds.

Mrs. Rosselini's breakdown had a powerful effect on how I viewed the complications of weight reduction. No longer were they episodes in a remote past, academic matters whose details had already slipped from the memory of my informants. These complications were now a burning problem.

I started to study them, even while putting the final touches on my paper, "The Night-Eating Pattern."

This paper was published in the respected *American Journal of Medicine*.[7] It described the night-eating pattern as consisting of over-eating in the evening and at night, agitation and insomnia, and then the morning lack of appetite. The pattern was present in 20 of our Medicine A obese patients and in none of 38 non-obese patients. Patients showing the pattern had great difficulty losing weight and paid a high price for trying. The conclusion stated that the pattern represents a special kind of response to stress, peculiar to some obese people, and that it is intimately bound up with their obesity.

Although I was eager to get on with my study of the responses to dieting, I paused to reflect on some of the lessons this study of the night-eating pattern had taught me. It was very different from the kind of research derived from the glucostatic theory. In that case, I had first deduced and then tested some consequences of a powerful theory. The tests had led to the discovery of new facts which helped to validate the theory. Here I had started with no theory at all, just an assumption—as Harold Wolff used to put it, in his characteristically intense manner, that "there is order in the universe." By the careful study of patients, and an unlikely event which called my attention to it, I had discerned a pattern in their behavior. Who could say where it would lead?

As with the work on the glucostatic theory, there was no simple outcome that would free obese people from their bondage. Although the night-eating seemed clearly related to stress, and was relieved with alleviation of the stress, this happy outcome was all too infrequent. It sometimes seemed as if the patients were worse off than before we had started.

But at least we had one more handle on the problem, and I pushed on, hoping that one day we would be able to do better.

four

Dieting and Depression

My first two research efforts, dealing with the glucostatic theory and the night-eating pattern, had started from somewhat detached concerns—to test a theory and to give a talk. Not so the third effort. This one took off from a concrete and pressing problem: to learn about the kind of emotional disturbance which had afflicted Mrs. Rosselini when she had tried to lose weight. For I was beginning to hear about similar troubles from other obese people. If this were a danger, it was one we had to know about. I was concerned not only for myself, but for all of the other physicians treating obese people, lest we actually add to the heavy burdens they were already carrying.

As instructive as these first two research efforts had been, the results had been modest. Both the glucostatic theory and the night-eating pattern had made inroads toward understanding obesity, and that was a beginning. But the paths they cut were far from central. It was clearly time for a third endeavor.

This next study started with an article of faith: that there was a consistent pattern to the emotional upsets I had observed in some of my patients when they attempted to diet. Perhaps a treatment program would evolve from learning more about this pattern.

I began by utilizing the natural history approach, that is, spending a great deal of time with each of the 25 obese patients I was then treating, and trying to find out everything I could about their past experiences with dieting. I tried to learn how often each one had dieted, how long the diets had lasted, why they had been undertaken, how the patient felt during the diet, and why he or she had stopped—in short anything that might throw light on the kind of difficulty Mrs. Rosselini had encountered.

My questions about the night-eating pattern had already revealed that eight of the twenty-five patients had experienced an emotional upset when they dieted. But these emotional upsets didn't fit any of the standard diagnoses. Depression was present, but so were anxiety and fatigue and feelings of futility. It took time before one fact became conspicuous: the diet which had ushered in the emotional disturbance had not been undertaken casually. In each case, it had had profound implications for the patient; the expectations had far exceeded what might reasonably have been hoped for from a diet. In more than one instance these expectations had been inadvertently fostered by a physician, sometimes by me, sometimes by another. There was at least some small comfort in learning that Mrs. Rosselini's illness was not unprecedented, and that other physicians had similarly blundered.

One patient's illness was particularly interesting, since I knew her physician and was able to compare his recollection of events with hers. (He had had no idea that his patient had become ill while dieting, and was stunned to learn of the part he had played.)

Maria Malone was a 34-year-old housewife who weighed 214 pounds when she came to Medicine A, complaining of obesity and migraine headaches. Her obesity had been slowly increasing since her adolescence, except for two attempts at weight reduction. The first attempt had been uneventful, the second disastrous, ushering in a severe emotional disturbance.

Mrs. Malone was the eldest of two daughters, raised in an authoritarian Irish-immigrant family. Much of her childhood had been spent in useless competition with her younger sister, who had become their parents' favorite because of her sickly childhood, her conforming behavior, and her supposedly greater abilities. After graduating from high school, Mrs. Malone had made an unsuccessful attempt to study art and then had become a secretary in a large industrial organization. There she had formed a strong attachment to a fellow worker. He must have been a curious man—bitter, rebellious, remarkably passive, 12 years her senior. She had idolized him throughout five years of a platonic friendship. And when he finally proposed marriage, she accepted at once, thrilled by this proposal and grateful to him for his motives for marrying her. He was willing to marry her, he announced, out of pure altruism. His goal was to develop her potential and to make her over into the wonderful person he was sure she could become.

As could have been forecast, their illusions did not survive the first months of marriage. They soon bogged down in a life of intense mutual dependency, bitter with recriminations about the supposedly inadequate care each was giving the other. Mrs. Malone gave birth to three children and raised them while going about her housewifely duties "as blank as that wall." Periodically she would break away into exuberant participation in community activities.

She had been worried for some years by the apparent attraction between her sister and her husband. One day she returned home to find them locked in a passionate embrace. Her immediate reaction was, "the world is falling apart," and she became panicky and disorganized. Her husband and sister, upset and chastened, made every effort to reassure Mrs. Malone about their love for her and the casualness of their relationship. But she was inconsolable. A week or two later, having assured herself that her husband and children were in the next room, she turned on the gas in the kitchen.

At this point her husband became alarmed and took her to the leading physician in the area, reputedly a wise and compassionate man. From what I knew about him this reputation was fully justified. Mrs. Malone was impressed, as others had been before her, by his kindness and understanding. She left his office after her first visit feeling much better. During her second visit, when he had learned more about the situation, he recommended that she return for weekly talks to help her understand some of her difficulties. When she protested that the family could not afford the expense, he replied that he would be willing to see her without charge. Puzzled, she asked him how this was possible. His reply, which loomed larger in later events, burned into her memory: "I'll be getting as much out of this as you."

At the time this doctor was becoming interested in psychotherapy and was selecting a few of his more articulate and troubled patients for regular interviews. Later, when I asked him about these events, he vaguely remembered having offered Mrs. Malone free weekly visits, but he had been quite unaware of the significance this offer had held for her. She came to his office once a week for about two months, and then stopped. She said she found she was, for no apparent reason, unable to talk to him. By this time she was over the acute anxiety and, so she thought, "back to my old self."

Several weeks after Mrs. Malone stopped seeing the doctor, she again had a sudden upset. It occurred when a neighbor brought up the subject of adultery. Mrs. Malone found herself becoming confused and excited. Unsure of what was happening to her, she hurriedly left her neighbor to try to straighten out her thoughts. These thoughts began to converge on one topic: a love affair with the doctor. As she went back over her talks with him, his remark, "I'll be getting as much out of this as you," began to assume a special meaning. Perhaps, she imagined, he had just been too shy to come right out and tell her his intentions. If that were the case, she decided to give him the opportunity. She called for another appointment.

But as soon as Mrs. Malone entered the doctor's office, her courage failed her. She became embarrassed and was unable to tell him why she had come. In fact, she had trouble saying anything. For a time the physician tried fruitlessly to help her to talk. Then, drumming his fingers on the table, he noted that she had not had a physical examination for some time. He suggested that it might be well to see how she was doing, and then proceeded to examine her. For Mrs. Malone the examination was a confirmation of all her hopes. Here was a man too shy to express his desires in a forthright way. But through his actions he left no doubt about his intentions. She returned home in high spirits.

When I spoke with the physician about these events, he vaguely remembered what had happened. He had been impressed first with Mrs. Malone's highly articulate account of her problems, and later with her growing difficulty in talking. He remembered feeling some relief when she had stopped coming for treatment, since things had been going so slowly. He did recall carrying out the physical examination, but none of the circumstances surrounding it, and learned of her reaction with the greatest chagrin.

For the next six months Mrs. Malone walked on air. Despite the fact that she did not see the physician during this time, she felt that "emotionally he was always with me, no matter where I was or what I did . . . It made me feel full, a terrible, pleasant sense of fullness." Much of her time was spent in romantic fantasies of how the doctor would come to rescue her from her drab and meaningless existence. In her mind, the physical examination had been not only an inarticulate expression of his sexual desire, but evidence as well of his wish that she become more attractive by losing weight. Exuberantly, and without the slightest difficulty, Mrs. Malone embarked on a reducing diet that brought her weight down from 225 to 175 pounds in less than six months.

During this period she seemed to have limitless energy, sailing through her formerly burdensome household activities with feelings of delight and accomplishment. She increased her participation in community activities and even resumed her old adolescent interest in painting. "It was different from the way things had been before. I had real feelings—love, and hate, and envy, and lust and passion." And for several weeks she luxuriated in her fantasies, with no concrete idea of when her rescue was to take place. She formed a vague notion that it would occur when her dieting had made her into the beautiful woman the physician's physical examination had revealed as the object of his desire. This notion became more concrete as her weight continued to melt away.

Then Mrs. Malone became troubled. With increasing apprehension she watched her weight decline towards the limit that would signal the transformation of her fantasy into reality. By the time it had reached 175 pounds, she could no longer keep her ideas to herself. With many misgivings, she gave her husband a much modified account of what she thought had been happening between her and the doctor.

Mr. Malone was furious. Exploding into a barrage of oaths, he dragged his wife out to their car and drove recklessly to the physician's office. Striding past the patients in the waiting area, he burst into the examining room with Mrs. Malone in his wake, shook his finger at the physician and told him in a loud dramatic voice never to see his wife again. Then, sulking and silent, he took her out of the office and drove home.

Dazed but relieved, Mrs. Malone spent the next day ruminating over the events of the confrontation—her husband's anger, the doctor's bewilderment, and her own sense of having been nothing more than a bystander. She finally satisfied herself that she had given her husband ample warning. She could now proceed without guilt or fear of recrimination. She telephoned the doctor and began by saying that she had been thinking about her husband's reaction. Then she added that perhaps he was right and that it might be better if they did not meet again. To her surprise the doctor agreed.

"I felt devastated, as if the most wonderful person in the world had died. It was a terrible sense of loss." For weeks she suffered from what she described as "emptiness," and her ebullient overactivity gave way to indolence and apathy. She lost interest in her personal appearance, kept wearing the same old black dress long after it had become dirty and wrinkled. She even stopped wearing make-up, and neglected her hair. Household chores again overwhelmed her. She could feed the children and get them off to school; and that was all.

As Mrs. Malone recovered from the initial shock of disillusionment, she began to be oppressed by "guilt," by "a horror of what I had been ready to do." This horror was intensified as she came to realize that the whole affair might have existed solely in her imagination. For months she languished in a state of morbid introspection, contemplating her depravity, "feeling I was wrong again, like I always used to be." It was the end of a year before most of these symptoms had subsided, and once again Mrs. Malone was back to her old, drab life. Her weight gradually increased to 225 pounds.

As I reviewed the emotional illnesses of my obese patients, it became clear not only that they were closely connected with a diet, but also that the diet had a special significance, closely related to attempts to achieve independence. Here was the same kind of conflict, between the desire for independence and the fear of it, which had loomed so large in the life of Maxine Wilkins. The diet, it appeared, gained its heightened significance as a symbol of independence; to diet and become thin was to become free. And the diets that portended trouble seemed to be those that coincided with a decision to break off an important dependency relationship.

If these assessments were even partially correct, they suggested certain precautions it would be well to take in treating Mrs. Malone. Her past history showed that she was vulnerable to dieting and to misinterpreting her relationship with a physician. She was also very dependent upon her husband, despite her denials and despite the bitterness of her complaints about him. I decided to support her efforts toward independence, but very cautiously.

Early in treatment both Mrs. Malone and I became aware of the dangers that faced us. She came to Medicine A at about the time that I was starting my systematic inquiry into the complications of dieting. We spent a good deal of time during her early visits in the clinic discussing these complications. We emerged from this inquiry with respect for the troubles that we could get into. But there were also some positive accomplishments. Talking about her illness seemed to help Mrs. Malone. Until then she had been unable to·think about it with any objectivity and instead had viewed it as an ominous period of confusion and chaos. She seemed to gain strength from discussing the illness, getting clear on just what had happened, on the chronology of events, on the limits of her guilt. One of the major benefits of psychotherapy for someone who has undergone a mental illness may be this simple one, of helping to bring order out of chaos, of getting clear with another person on just what did happen.

The next step was to help Mrs. Malone express her anger towards her husband and to help her understand why she felt so angry. Then, very cautiously, we attempted to help her take some small, realistic steps toward greater independence. By consolidating her many community activities, for instance, she was able to take on greater responsibility in those she chose to continue.

One of my major goals in treating Mrs. Malone was to stay out of trouble. This was certainly a come-down from the grand goals of a few years before. In psychoanalytic training our greatest scorn had been reserved for what we called "melioristic" approaches to treatment. Nothing less than thorough-going personality reorganization would satisfy us as a worthy goal. And now here I was adopting a melioristic approach if ever there was one. And it seemed quite appropriate.

Over a period of a year and a half we succeeded in staying out of trouble. She lost some weight, from the 214 pounds which she brought to Medicine A to 190 pounds. Her migraine headaches stopped almost completely. And when we finally terminated treatment, it was for a reason I had never expected. *Mr.* Malone became ill. As his wife showed a slow but steady increase in her ability to manage her affairs, and she became less dependent upon him, Mr. Malone became frightened, then angry. He finally developed a peptic ulcer. In time the ulcer became unmanageable; and he was forced to spend longer and longer periods in the hospital.

The origins of this difficulty seemed clear, and Mrs. Malone and I spoke about it at length, trying to see how her increasing independence might be made less threatening to him. But he was not in a position to accept help from his wife. And he adamantly refused both her and my suggestions that he seek psychotherapy. So Mrs. Malone eventually gave up treatment and went back to a somewhat less driven dependency upon her husband. Mr. Malone recovered from his ulcer. And they went on—unhappy, still mutually recriminatory, but perhaps a bit more comfortable than before.

This was my most impressive experience with the interlocking neuroses of marital partners. It was not to be the last. I feel sure, from the vantage point of today's knowledge about family therapy, that a great deal more could have been done for the Malones had I felt free to treat Mr. Malone along with his wife. I believe he might have welcomed this kind of help, which he could have seen as a way of rehabilitating his sick wife. And small shifts in the equilibrium of the two might well have accomplished as much for their adjustment as a major personality reorganization of Mrs. Malone would have. For then she would not have been forced to choose between living with a disconsolate husband or abandoning him.

But the teaching of the day frowned upon a psychiatrist treating both husband and wife. And it disparaged the results of such treatment as "superficial . . . environmental manipulation, . . . mere social work." So I did what I had been taught to do, and learned more about the inadequacy of our methods. This learning was to serve me in good stead in my treatment of Phyllis Baker.

Of all the patients who taught me about dieting and depression, Phyllis Baker stands out as my best teacher. Like Maria Malone, she had undergone a severe emotional illness during an earlier attempt at dieting. As with Maria Malone, I started treatment well aware of the possible dangers and took particular care to avoid them. What happened thus seems particularly significant.

Phyllis Baker was one of the most obese patients I had yet treated. Only five feet tall, she weighed 240 pounds when she arrived at Medicine A to say that her eating was out of control and her weight increasing rapidly. Her appearance was remarkable. She was a woman of 22 years, who appeared to be in her middle teens. Her enormous body was covered by a dirty, cheap, cotton print dress that was stained and wrinkled. Perched atop this mammoth body, her small and striking head was dominated by a large aquiline nose and a mass of unkempt, red-blonde hair which swept out from her head in an untidy mass. On what must have been the apex of her massive breasts, two buttons advertised the Liberal Party candidate for mayor in the forthcoming election.

Phyllis was obviously very anxious as I invited her to sit down. Her hands were in almost constant motion, and she kept wringing them in the motion of distress of women three times her age. When she spoke her voice quavered and broke. She was barely able to tell me why she had come to the clinic.

Obesity was only one of her problems. Equally serious, she felt, was her problem with alcohol. She spent almost every evening in bars, drank to drunkenness every other night, and found herself in all manner of distasteful and dangerous circumstances as a result. She also said she was very nervous in crowds or groups of people. Her appearance made all this quite believable.

As Phyllis unfolded her many problems, I began to share her sense of being overwhelmed. Yet she had been working, supporting herself, getting by. She must have had some hope that she could be helped. "What," I asked, "do you hope to get out of treatment?"

She didn't hesitate. "To become a worthwhile member of the human race." I said that I gathered she did not feel that way now. She replied, "I feel the farthest thing from it."

The desolation and horror chilled me. "How *do* you feel about yourself?"

Again she did not hesitate. "I think of myself as a great mass of gray-green, amorphous material. Then at times I feel like a sloth. And just now, when I got up on the examining table, I felt like an elephant."

I had rarely heard anyone, even patients hospitalized for mental illness, condemn themselves with the intensity of Phyllis Baker. She felt that people were watching her. Perhaps they really were; perhaps she just imagined it. But the self-loathing accorded fully with her complaint that things seemed unreal much of the time. Her account was as unsettling as her appearance.

Phyllis Baker's memories of childhood were marked by almost unrelieved gloom. She was one of several illegitimate children, who, with an older brother, had been left in the care of a widow, whom she had come to know as "Mother." She had few memories before those of her first day at school. Soon after she arrived, still excited by the occasion, she was picked out of her class by the school nurse, who found lice in her hair and dutifully announced the fact to the class. She was sent home with a note to her mother to wash her hair in kerosene.

Many children have been concerned by what the neighbors think of their family. For Phyllis, the problem was what the vice squad thought. When she was seven years old, the vice squad took a special interest in the "rooming house" which was her mother's ostensible source of income. Their concern was for the moral influence on the children. The problem was "solved" by getting her mother to marry one of the "boarders," a quiet and ineffectual man. Phyllis said, "When I found out about this, I was overwhelmed by his generosity and goodness. He just did it for me. He didn't have any other reason. The marriage was never consum-

mated." It was only later, while she was in treatment, that
Phyllis discovered that this was not the case, and her disillusionment increased.

Phyllis' own sexual experiences began at age five, when
she thought she had had sexual intercourse with a boy. She
knew that she had had intercourse by age six, for her sex play
was with teenage boys, ". . . and it hurt terribly when they
got into me." By then she had been discovered by her brother,
who kept threatening to tell her mother. She had spent sleep-
less nights wondering what was going to happen to her, and
remembered lying in bed waiting for her heart to stop beating.

Twelve was a critical age for Phyllis, the year when her
periods started, and fear of pregnancy stopped her sexual
activity. She had looked forward to this time, hoping that
abstinence might make her more comfortable. The opposite
had occurred. The severe, sometimes crippling anxiety that
had struck me so forcibly during our first meeting had begun
then. It was present only some of the time, but the fact that
it began at a time that she had hoped would bring an end
to her fearfulness had been profoundly disillusioning. She had
begun to over-eat, and had become obese.

We spent a great deal of time trying to understand her
over-eating and the period when it had begun. She felt that
part of the explanation lay in the family's attitude toward
food. "They always impressed on me as a child that if you
eat, you are secure. That's one sign of security. I remembered
so often my father saying, 'Well, we'll never starve. We've
always got food on the table.' I suppose that's why I get so
much pleasure out of food, and why I feel so strong when
I'm eating."

At times Phyllis insisted that she did not over-eat because
of hunger. She had feelings that others might interpret as
hunger—like emptiness in the upper part of her abdomen—but
she didn't consider this hunger. "It's emptiness, just general
emptiness, and it goes away completely when I eat." It was
always hard for me to believe that her feelings of emptiness
in the abdomen differed from what other people called hunger.

But her eating experiences certainly differed. "It's like I'm in love with food when I'm eating." Afterwards she felt remorse. "When I finish, I really hate food. After I've eaten, lost of times I feel sick. But when I'm eating, I feel good."

When Phyllis had begun to over-eat, at age 12, it was mostly during the day. But by the time she began treatment she was in the night-eating pattern, which was unusual in view of the large amounts of alcohol she consumed and the various foods available in bars.

The age of 12 had been memorable also for "the big family split." For some time a boarder, not her father, had tried to take on the disciplining of Phyllis' increasingly delinquent brother. Eventually the boarder's beatings led to violent arguments between Phyllis' mother and father, which culminated in a fight, during which her mother knocked her father down. Bitterly the family split into two factions, Phyllis, her mother, and the boarder in one, her father and brother in the other. They divided the house into halves, and for years thereafter the members of each faction religiously stayed in their assigned part of the house.

Despite the enormous difficulties under which she labored, Phyllis had done surprisingly well in her school work. As graduation from high school had approached, she had begun to look upon college as an escape from her trouble-ridden home. When her application to a nearby junior college was accepted, she was elated and joyfully prepared to leave home. Her mother's response was uncompromising opposition. Ordinary work was good enough for most people; why did Phyllis feel above it? She might as a starter, her mother suggested, begin to repay all the sacrifices she had made for a daughter who was not even hers. When gentler measures did not suffice, her mother began to berate Phyllis for her arrogance and cruelty in presuming to set herself above the family.

But Phyllis went nonetheless; and the first few weeks away from home were exciting ones. She embarked on a series of self-improvement measures, prominent among them her first serious attempt at dieting. In six months she lost 70 pounds.

What happened thereafter never became very clear. The work she undertook to support herself took time away from her school assignments. School was much harder than she had expected. Her classmates were no more friendly than they had been in high school. She failed her mid-year exams. Six months after leaving home Phyllis returned, frightened and defeated.

She said that she had suffered at that time from a "minor depression," and preferred not to talk about it. But what she did say revealed no "minor" depression. For a year and a half she had been unable to work. She stayed home, crying, depressed, unconcerned about her appearance—feeling futile, apathetic, and without hope. She regained the weight she had lost, and with a measure of relief, surrendered the conduct of her life to her mother.

The results were not quite what she expected. Accepting Phyllis as a colleague, her mother took her along on nightly rounds of pub-crawling. Life was soon dominated by heavy drinking and sex. Neither was satisfying. For Phyllis a drinking bout was precipitated by feelings quite different from the sense of "emptiness" that started her eating. "Rage," and to a lesser extent "frustration" were ". . . what started me drinking. When I get started with a bottle, I have a wonderful feeling of defiance. The hell with the whole world. I don't need anybody or anything, and nobody can do a damned thing to me. Screw 'em all."

Phyllis had been about 16 when she first became aware of a new kind of problem, new feelings that were later to cause her great distress. They began as romantic fantasies. "I would spend all of my time in my room, just lying there and thinking about being a man. I would be a sailor and travel all over the world. Or I would be a famous card player and go to Monte Carlo, and play cards, and rescue a damsel in distress. Particularly, most of all, I wanted to be a famous pitcher in the big leagues." Often the daydreams were quite focused. "I wanted a penis. I wanted to be a tall, dark, handsome man with a penis."

Phyllis had bridged the gap from fantasy to action in the sexual sphere, as in many others, with alcohol. All she had to do was to be present in a bar, in the security of the half-light, get drunk, and let things happen. She would be picked up by a woman and taken off, with no initiative on her part. Then, when the love-making started, "I come alive. I remember so well the first time. Afterwards I felt so proud . . . gay . . . light-hearted . . . responsible." There was no similarity to the fearful, furtive sex with men. Here was real excitement, ". . . the excitement of giving of myself, of making love, of giving love. I adore being allowed to play the male part."

We discussed at length what it meant to love women and how she had felt about it. "No, I don't feel like a man then, even though I do feel like I'm doing a man's work. I feel I have to satisfy the women." And she ruminated over male and female, man and woman. "It's not like being a man, and it's not like being a woman. I guess it sounds kind of wacky, but what it's really like is a boy doing a man's work."

Once, many months into treatment, Phyllis began to talk about her sexual feelings with increased intensity. It was quite important, somehow, to tell me about them. At first she could not, but finally she said, "I'm not sure about wanting to take care of other women. I think that's all too noble. I just want to get my head in between her legs. That's what gives me real peace! Being walled off, and walled in, and restful."

Gradually, as the months passed and Phyllis kept coming to the clinic, many of the terrible and often desperate concerns she expressed were supplanted by a theme which became the major issue in treatment, as it was in her life. This was her long-standing bitter quarrel with her mother. It was somehow linked to what seemed an almost irresistible need on Phyllis's part to return to her mother's home each weekend. She had no idea why she kept going back, particularly since she always seemed to have such a terrible time. In fact, she usually found herself drinking, even drunk, before arriving home. And she frequently stayed drunk most of the weekend.

Over the months we worked on this theme of Phyllis' need to return to mother, and over the months her anger towards her mother grew. I had seldom heard such venomous hatred as that which wracked her after her weekends at home. And it was almost as if the more she hated the more she needed to return. But why?

As we talked it became clearer. Going home was a way of reassuring herself that she had not hurt her mother by what she said about her in treatment; but it was more than that. When she allowed her mother to humiliate and degrade her, she assured herself not only that she had not hurt her mother, but that she could not hurt her. By going home, and getting drunk, and sleeping with men, she was in effect saying, "See, I'm not really defying you by running off to New York. I'm not trying to set myself over you. I'm really just like you in every miserable, bad way."

As she reached this understanding Phyllis became calm, even radiant. She announced that she had decided to be nice to herself for a change, and she looked it. She was wearing an attractive new dress, and a new coat and lipstick that set off her beautiful blue eyes. Her unruly hair was set in the first permanent wave she had ever had. She was through with the penitent trips home, she reported, and had told her mother that she would not be back the following weekend, or for the Thanksgiving holidays the week after that. She did not seem elated. But she had started a diet and lost nine pounds in a week . . .

This good fortune did not last long. Phyllis called the following week to say that she could not keep her appointment. Later I learned what had happened. Things had continued to go wonderfully well for the six days after her last visit to the clinic. Then on the morning of her next visit she had awakened in a panic after a vivid, terrifying dream:

"I am back in my home town in a telephone booth, and I am about to have a baby. My father and brother came, and I have the baby. It is very realistic, pains and everything. The cord is there, and I don't know what to do with it. My father kneels down and begins gnawing on it like a rat. It hurts. I am very frightened and start screaming. Then he bites through it. I woke up terrified."

Phyllis said that she knew that the dream was about ". . . my fear of leaving home. The umbilical cord is what binds me to my parents. I am terribly afraid of having it cut."

She had bounded out of bed after the dream, shaking, jittery, tense. The feelings mounted to unbearable anxiety. When she began to shake all over, she found herself debating whether this was a shaking chill which meant that she had pneumonia, or whether it was simply fear, in which case she was surely going insane. She decided on pneumonia: "It was serious and physical, and would explain why I felt so awful." Leaving her apartment early in the morning, she rushed home.

Phyllis greeted her astonished mother with the report that she was deathly ill and in desperate need of help. "And just as soon as I was there, I felt much better. I just went to bed and let Mother feed me, and I ate and ate and ate." By the end of the week she had regained the nine pounds, and her anxiety was decreasing.

The following week, having bolstered her courage with "a few drinks," Phyllis left home to keep her appointment with me. Glumly she told me what had happened. She spoke about being afraid of me and afraid of coming in to see me. "We have talked a lot about my hatred for my mother, but we've neglected my need for her. We just ignored that, and I need her terribly." I agreed.

For a month she continued to be tense and frightened during the day, and drunk at night. The old feeling that people were watching her returned with unprecedented severity. As we were walking into the office, she looked around her in such a frightened, trapped way that I asked if she were afraid of being in the office. She said that she was, but it wasn't just my office; she looked around her this way all the time now. She told me of spending every free hour at home with

her mother. Usually she felt better there, and she complained
that she couldn't understand why. "The price of going back
is my self-respect. You can't have any idea of how bad it
is there, everyone yelling all the time, Mother heckling me
for everything I do. Someone is always yelling, 'Do this, do
that' . . . 'I'll break your arm if you don't stop that' . . . 'I'll
knock your teeth out if you don't do that!' "

As the months went by, however, Phyllis became less
frightened. She no longer felt that people were watching her,
and she no longer gave the impression of feeling trapped when
she was in my office. On the other hand, she became increasingly morose and sad. Her communications were sparse and
hostile. For long periods she would sit silently, responding
to my questions and comments solely with gestures, or not
at all. Then she began to break her appointments, and I found
it harder and harder to keep track of what was happening
in her life. Clearly she was drinking heavily, and borrowing
to pay for it. Her alcoholism was interfering with her work,
her friendships, her treatment, and ultimately, her life.

One morning I was awakened by the telephone ringing,
to hear a weak voice saying, "I've slashed my wrists." In
fact she had, but the bleeding had stopped by the time I
reached her, and she bitterly handed me her blood-caked
suicide note. It read in part: "I've got to be punished because
I am a monster inside, all ugly and creepy, and I'll never
be any different." She had carried out part of the punishment
she felt she needed by cutting a deep "H" into her arm,
". . . to brand myself as a homosexual." Now exhausted, all tension and anxiety gone, she just wanted to go to bed and rest.

This crisis passed, as had others. But both of us realized
that what we were doing was not enough. Ten months after
her last ill-fated attempt at dieting, with treatment at a stand-
still and her life going downhill, Phyllis entered a mental
hospital.

Its doctors took complete care of her, and I saw Phyllis
only infrequently when I went as a visitor. But these visits,
and talks with her psychiatrist, gave me a good picture of
her course in the hospital. The treatment program helped

her a great deal. She took part in a wide variety of hospital activities. When she left the hospital after ten months, she was considerably improved. During her hospital stay, she also had gone on a diet.

This diet is worthy of note. She began it soon after her admission, when she was still quite depressed; she continued it until her discharge. And she lost more weight than during any of her previous diets, 80 pounds. She weighed 275 on admission and 195 at discharge. How did this weight loss affect her emotionally? It did not have the devastating consequences of her earlier ones. She did not undergo another period of panic and disorganization like the one that had marked the onset of her illness in Medicine A. In fact, she became much less depressed.

What conclusion did I draw from this experience at dieting? For one, Phyllis was able for the first time in her life to lose a large amount of weight without becoming depressed. It seems reasonable to believe that this favorable outcome was due to the active treatment and support she received in the hospital. She was anxious and tense during this time, but no more so than usual.

In my mind I began to separate the ill effects from dieting into two categories: psychological and biological. For Phyllis, Mrs. Rosselini, and Mrs. Malone, psychological factors seemed to play a central role in their dieting depressions. Dieting and weight loss, the symbols of freedom and independence, and the subsequent difficulties of living with this freedom, were too prominent to ignore. But biological factors, the effects of food deprivation, may well have increased their vulnerability to the psychological conflicts. Certainly non-specific results of weight reduction, such as irritability and tension, could affect the obese as well as the non-obese.

I treated Phyllis for two years after her discharge from the hospital, until I moved away from New York. And I kept in touch with her for several years after that. The most important development in her life was to join Alcoholics Anonymous. When I last heard from her, she had been sober for eight years. Her performance at work had improved as soon as she stopped drinking, and she gradually rose to a responsible position in a large company. After considerable sexual experimentation with men and women, and much associated turmoil, she had accepted her homosexuality and had been living relatively happily with another woman for some years. She had been able to keep her weight below 200 pounds. And she had achieved a dearly won sense of pride, and an ability to manage her life.

At this time very little had appeared in the medical literature about the complications of losing weight. Yet concern with obesity and weight reduction had been mounting until it had assumed the proportions of a national neurosis. The time seemed ripe for a report on the problem.

The first part of my report[8] dealt with the frequency of emotional disturbances during efforts at weight reduction. Among the vulnerable persons I had treated in Medicine A, nine of the first twenty-five had become disturbed while dieting. Four of these disturbances had occurred while I was treating them; eight others had occurred previously. (Three of the patients experienced two illnesses each, making a total of twelve illnesses in nine patients.)

The next part of the report described the illnesses themselves. They all had two distinct phases, characterized first by symptoms of anxiety, and later by those of depression. In addition, half the illnesses had been initiated by a period of mild elation, with some overactivity and increased feelings of well-being. The elation would begin at about the time the patient decided to break off an important dependency relationship, and was often first manifested by the feelings of exultation with which the patient celebrated his or her apparent freedom. These feelings were intensified by the decision to diet. Many of the patients had long cherished secret dreams of the extravagant benefits to be achieved by weight reduction, and when, after years of indecision, they sought to live out this fantasy, it was with excited anticipation. This heightened mood persisted for weeks and even months.

Typically the elation was abruptly terminated, by a short period of anxiety. Some apparently minor incident would bring home to the patients the consequences of the course they were following, and they would react with severe anxiety. During this time they would become preoccupied with the danger of living without the support they had so gratuitously cut off. And perhaps more importantly, the patients would begin to fear the retaliation of the authority they had defied.

Within a week or two anxiety would be displaced by a depressive reaction that might last for months. During this period the patients would feel generally depressed, with frequent crying spells and disturbed sleep. In each case the disorder was severe enough to interfere with the ability to work. Suicidal ruminations were common, but self-destructive attempts were rare.

Recovery occurred in all the patients after illnesses which lasted from six weeks to a year, but the factors leading to recovery were not clear. Although all the patients discontinued their reducing diets soon after the onset of severe symptoms, increased food intake did not terminate the illnesses. Furthermore, in each case the disrupted personal relationship was restored, but this could as easily have been a result of the recovery as a cause.

The report on the 25 patients was now complete. But they were a select group. Referred to Medicine A because of the severity of their obesity or difficulty in its management, they undoubtedly represented a high proportion of emotionally disturbed people. I didn't know whether this proportion was higher in this particular group than in the average severely obese group. The usefulness of the report to the practicing physician would be greatly increased if, in addition to providing information about these more difficult patients, I could say something about dieting by the average obese patient who comes to the family doctor. Specifically, how often do these patients develop such symptoms when they diet?

The nearest thing to a cross-section of dieters was the group of patients who came to the Nutrition Clinic of the New York Hospital. I had become well acquainted with this Clinic in the course of referring patients for reducing diets. It was an ideal place to study the average overweight dieter, for it treated a true cross-section of them. I was able to arrange for interviews of 100 patients.

Instead of trying to keep in touch with all 100 patients to find out how they tolerated their *present* reducing diets, we simply asked them about their *previous* diets. This method had the disadvantage of requiring patients to remember events that might be long forgotten. It was subject to the well-known retrospective falsification which can occur in such recall. Nevertheless, it allowed us to obtain information on 100 percent of our group of patients, an unusual record in the study of obese people. Furthermore, the process was very economical.

We were surprised by the results. 72 of the 100 patients had dieted previously, several of them on many occasions. Of these, 54 percent reported such symptoms as nervousness, weakness and irritability during at least one reducing regimen; and 55 percent of all such regimens were characterized by the presence of symptoms.

The report of this study on "The Dieting Depression"[8] was greeted with interest by many physicians. I was pleased by this interest because of the possibility that it might herald a change in their usual harsh attitudes toward such patients. Perhaps it might lead them to treat them with more respect. As early as medical school I had been aware of the condescending and punitive attitude of some doctors towards their obese patients. Even physicians who were relatively uncritical of them still found them frustrating, boring, irritating.

As my teaching had put me in contact with more and more practitioners, I had begun to sense that their negative attitudes were the result of two underlying assumptions: first, that weight reduction programs are effective, and second, that they are harmless. Compared with the more acute diseases with which physicians dealt, obesity seemed a trivial disorder. If, in addition, they thought that weight reduction was an easy matter, they might quite understandably be frustrated by the failure of their patients to lose weight.

By this time my own experience had convinced me that weight-reduction programs were not nearly as effective as was generally believed. And the "Dieting Depression" study in-

dicated that they might not be harmless. To my great satisfaction, physicians on the firing line seemed ready to accept
both these points. If their treatment of obese patients produced
results no worse than those of others, they had no reason to
blame themselves or to criticize their patients. And the idea
that a treatment might have adverse side reactions was a
well-recognized part of medical practice. The demonstration
that treatment for obesity could produce such ill effects tended
to legitimize the treatment *and* the condition toward which
treatment was directed. As a result physicians were increasingly able to see obesity as a respectable medical problem
and less as a sign of moral weakness. Respecting their patients'
problem made it easier to respect the patients themselves.

At times, however, I became concerned by an overly
enthusiastic endorsement of the idea that weight reduction
might have its hazards for obese people. For it could be used
to discourage any treatment of obesity. Such an attitude was
particularly distressing because evidence was accumulating
that weight reduction could have some very favorable effects
upon health.

One particularly significant study cited people who had
been refused life insurance because of obesity. They had then
lost weight and consequently qualified for life insurance. These
people showed far lower mortality rates than did obese people.
For the women in the study the mortality rate was as low
as if they had never been obese. These findings made it a
singularly inappropriate time to discourage all efforts at weight
reduction; and I was concerned that our study was being used
to support this negative point of view.

In the years following publication of "The Dieting Depression" many papers were published on the subject. Some
supported the view that there was little if any correlation
between depression and dieting; others supported my less
optimistic conclusions. Controversy grew as to whether dieting
made obese people feel better or worse. I became confused,
and I had to assume that others must be at least as confused.
How was the physician in practice to interpret these conflicting reports?

It was not until I sat down to write this book that I was finally able to resolve this conflict to my own satisfaction. For once I had the leisure to review the literature, it became apparent that most forms of dieting carried with them a high likelihood of emotional disturbance. And, paradoxically, the strongest evidence in support of this conclusion was provided by precisely those reports which denied the dangers of dieting. One, for example, reported symptoms in half the people undertaking reducing diets; another reported premature discontinuation by 75 per cent. These dismal figures applied not only to the more lenient diets of people living at home, but even to the carefully supervised long-term diets in hospitals.[9]

And there, for the time being, the matter of dieting and depression rests. It has left us with respect for the difficulties of dieting, and that is to the good. Obese people need all the understanding they can get. And it has not precluded efforts at weight reduction by those people who must lose weight for medical, as opposed to cosmetic, reasons. Finally, it has given us a baseline against which to measure new methods of treatment for obesity. If a new treatment is as effective as, or more effective than, the old ones, and if it does not produce as much emotional difficulty, clearly it has much to recommend it. And such a treatment may well be at hand, as we shall see in Chapter 10.

five
Binge-Eating

An invitation to give a talk at a psychiatric hospital in New York stimulated my next endeavor—an inquiry which defined a second eating pattern, the eating binge. This inquiry did not start from observations about patients, as had the study of night eating, but rather from new information about brain mechanisms, derived from experiments with animals. The discovery of brain areas which control eating was still fresh, and we had not yet fully assimilated the unexpected finding that there were not one but two pairs of such areas. One triggers eating and the other inhibits it. Why this division of labor?

The idea that there are brain areas that stimulate eating was not surprising; such areas had been postulated long before their discovery. What was a surprise was the discovery of satiety areas which inhibit eating. For traditionally, satiety had been viewed as a purely incidental aspect of eating—what happened when the drive to eat ran out of steam. But if that were all there is to satiety, separate brain areas to inhibit eating would be quite unnecessary. Yet satiety areas existed, and their destruction was followed promptly by over-eating and obesity. Furthermore, the over-eating which followed destruction of the satiety areas had some strange and unexpected characteristics.

For example, if rats with their satiety areas destroyed were allowed free access to food, they over-ate in an uncontrolled manner, often consuming twice their usual amount of food, as if all the brakes had been removed. But when any obstruction was placed in their way, their food intake fell not only below its usual level, but even below that of non-obese rats faced with a similar obstruction. It made no difference what form the obstruction took, whether it involved lifting heavy covers to reach the food, solving mazes, pressing levers, electric shocks, even adulteration with quinine. Faced with such impediments, the obese rats simply sat down on the job and ate *less* than non-obese rats under the same circumstances.

This research exploded traditional views of "hunger" as a unitary phenomenon. Hunger as defined by how much food an animal eats is apparently quite different from hunger as defined by how hard the animal will work to obtain food.

These experiments with animals also had a liberating effect upon our understanding of the way obese people eat. We were no longer forced to account for all over-eating in terms of increased hunger (although that could, of course, still be the case). We now knew that over-eating might also result from decreased satiety, and that these two forms of over-eating might well differ dramatically.

The night-eating pattern seemed a classic instance of over-eating as a failure of satiety—for a characteristic complaint of night-eaters was an inability to stop eating once they started. They rarely spoke of being hungry. Instead, I heard time and again how difficult it was to stop eating as long as food was available, how they found themselves nibbling and just could not seem to stop. Yet if food were not available, they rarely developed any strong desire to eat or made any great effort to obtain food. Even when severely agitated, they would rarely so much as leave the house to buy food.

So much for over-eating due to failure of satiety. What about over-eating due to an increased hunger drive? Did it occur in humans as well as in experimental animals? The question kept coming back more and more insistently. So I set about searching for obese people who described their over-eating in terms suggestive of increased hunger. I soon met a promising candidate.

Hyman Cohen was a 37-year-old high school teacher referred to me by a mutual friend. This friend said that Mr. Cohen was a "compulsive eater," and his description of this eating made it sound as if it might be due to an increased hunger drive. The description intrigued me. So did another aspect: the possibility of intensive treatment of an obese man. I had already come to realize how infrequently men seek treatment for their obesity. Of the 25 obese patients who served as subjects for the night-eating study, only two were men. And I knew neither well.

From the moment that Hyman Cohen walked through the door, it was clear that he was quite different from the passive, obese women with whom I had grown so familiar. A big, burly man with large shoulders and a massive chest, he strode into the office, rolling as the very obese must because of the thickness of their thighs. And the girth of his upper arms forced his arms out from his sides, something in the manner of a wrestler. He was clearly obese—carrying 272 pounds on his five-foot-nine frame—but the impression that he gave was not what I had come to expect from my experiences with obese women. He had tremendous vitality and vigor.

Mr. Cohen shook my hand with a bone-crunching grasp; later I learned that he spent a great deal of time in weight-lifting and body building exercises. Even when he sat down,

uncomfortably bulging out of the chair and bursting out of
his clothing, he still seemed forceful and aggressive. His face
was round and full, his eyes slits behind large horn-rimmed
glasses, his head covered with short, brown, curly hair. He
began speaking at once and continued at length, almost without interruption. His speech was booming and forceful. He
punctuated his remarks with frequent outbursts of laughter,
at first nervous and shy, but eventually loud and even raucous.
At times he spoke of what he called his "Rabelaisian" activities—and it seemed to me, as I sat listening silently to his
flood of speech, that Rabelaisian was a fitting description of
his entire appearance and manner.

Mr. Cohen got to the point at once. The immediate
stimulus for his coming to see me was that he was being
considered for the position of principal at the high school
where he taught. He wanted the job because it meant a
substantial salary increase. But he now weighed over 270
pounds and could not pass the required physical examination.
He had six months to reduce, and if he were successful, he
was certain that he would not only pass the physical but get
the job.

"So, I want you to peel this weight off and get me down
to fighting shape."

Mr. Cohen went on to say that he had a problem with
biting his fingernails and help up his hands to show nails
bitten to the quick, pink, tender skin bulging out about them,
and traces of what appeared to be clotted blood in the depressions at the bottom of the nails. He also reported that he
was always in debt. He thought his indebtedness, his nail-bit-
ing, and his obesity were somehow connected, but he was
not sure how.

He beamed proudly as he told me of this connection
and went on to say that he knew a great deal about himself.
He had been, he explained, "psychoanalyzed" four or five
years before. It developed that he had seen a psychoanalyst
for treatment at that time, going twice a week for about a
year. He said that it had been a resounding success, that it
had cleared up all of his emotional problems and had left

him with deep insights, not only into himself but also into those around him.

He counted his "psychoanalysis" as one of the most important experiences in his life, if not *the* most important. Although he had not had any serious emotional problems before the treatment, it had, he said, left him in a state of perfect contentment. He went on to describe his happy marriage, his lovely son, his challenging job. I had become accustomed to hearing obese people tell me in our first interview how well their lives were going. But I had never encountered a tale of such utter bliss.

Finally, about forty minutes after he entered the office, Mr. Cohen began to run down a bit. I was then able to put into words my mounting doubts. "If things are going so well," I asked, "why are you coming to see me?"

Brought up sharply, Mr. Cohen paused and looked quizzically at me. "For psychotherapy, of course."

I admitted my bewilderment. "Why?"

Mr. Cohen replied in a tone of voice that implied any damn fool ought to know the answer to that one: "Well, obesity *is* a psychosomatic problem, isn't it?"

I hesitated. Despite the countless things he had already told me about himself, I had the feeling that I did not know this man at all. And I was increasingly puzzled about what it was he wanted of me. Finally I began slowly: "Yes . . . People do consider obesity a psychosomatic disease . . . But it must have a number of different causes. . . ." I floundered along, discomfited by his growing and very apparent disappointment.

For a time neither of us said anything. Then I tried again. "Well, what puzzles me is, your life seems to be going along very well. You haven't told me about any problems. . . ."

"Just the obesity. That's right. I don't have any problems except for the obesity. That's what I'm here for, to get it cleared up."

"But you say that you don't have any problems, no worries or conflicts that might be causing the obesity . . ." I ventured.

"That's right," he replied. "Emotions are definitely not involved. There is no connection there. I haven't had any emotional problems since my psychoanalysis."

"Well, then, why . . ." I began, and then I stopped. Our time was up, and I welcomed relief from this perplexing encounter. Perhaps we could do better next time. I told Mr. Cohen I did not feel I had yet gotten a grasp on the problem. Would he like to come back next week at the same time?

"I certainly would, doctor, I'll be here. You can count on that." He rose, crushed my hand with his vise-like grasp, and strode out the door.

I approached our next meeting with concern. What was it Mr. Cohen really wanted? How could I clarify it? What could I do about whatever it was that was bothering him? How was I to begin?

I needn't have worried. Mr. Cohen was waiting for me when I arrived at the office, strode in and seated himself with assurance and asked, "Well, doctor, where do we go from here? I feel that I want to do whatever I can to be a good experimental subject. I want to help your research in every possible way."

"Experimental subject?" I asked.

"Yes," he went on. "I've had a long talk with Mr. Leibowitz (the mutual friend who had referred him to me) about your research, and I want to do everything within my power to help it along."

I murmured feebly that I did not want him to think of himself as an experimental subject, that I considered our relationship as one of patient and doctor, and that I saw my job as trying to help him decide what difficulties he was having and what he might do about them. Not surprisingly, in view of my failure in that attempt during our last visit, Mr. Cohen appeared a bit crestfallen. "Don't you want to see me any more?" he pleaded.

Gamely trying to preserve the illusion that I was exploring the possibility of psychotherapy with him, I returned to our discussion of the previous week and said that I didn't think we had gotten clear on his problem.

He immediately assured me, "The problem is my obesity, and what the hell I am going to do about it. It's completely out of control. I've gained nearly 60 pounds in the last year and I'm eating all the time now. I've had this crazy idea '. . . Dr. Stunkard is going to take care of me. So I can do anything I want to, because when I get to him everything will be all right.' " He stopped and looked imploringly at me. "You've just got to help me."

Suddenly it all became clear. Beneath the bluster and bravado was a frightened man, desperately appealing for help. How could I have failed to see this?

The next step was easy. "O.K. How do we do it?"

"Well, as I see it," he began, his confidence returning, "it's all just a matter of will power. I can start a diet any time I want to. And I can lose a hell of a lot of weight when I am on one. But right now my will power just doesn't seem to be up to it. That's where you come in. It's like hiring a policeman to check on me. If I am going to have to face the scales each week, I am simply going to have to stop eating so much. It's as simple as that.

"Also it's a little like being a Catholic and going to confession. When I was going to see my analyst, I would confess my sins and then I would feel better. I got some release last week just telling you about my eating. I never talk to anyone else about it. It makes me think of *Crime and Punishment,* like the criminal who always has to talk about his crimes. There's another book about it, *Island in the Sun.* It has the same theme—the criminal with an implacable desire to tell of his crimes . . . to confess his sins."

Warming to the topic, he went on. Finally I said that I was impressed with the way he described himself as a criminal—as guilty of some crime because of his eating.

"Of course. This damned weight is not only damaging my job prospects but it's shortening my life expectancy. So, indirectly, it's going to hurt my wife as well as me."

I said that his talk sounded much more urgent than concern over job prospects and life expectancy. These seemed relatively abstract long-range considerations. He seemed, I insisted, to be talking about something much more urgent. What was it?

"My guilt drives me here," he said. "But why do I feel so guilty? Why is it so out of proportion to what I have done? It's not that terrible to over-eat and yet I feel it is."

"Do you have any idea why it seems so terrible?" I asked.

"I just don't know. I just don't have any idea. It's just that this eating has become an obsession with me. I think about it all the time. It's the first thing I think of when I wake up in the morning and it's the last thing I think of when I go to bed at night." As Mr. Cohen talked on, he kept referring to his eating. Food kept coming into the conversation with a persistence that amazed me. Almost everything he talked about had to do with food. I had never heard anything like it.

He told of a time when he had thought that his eating might be an attempt to obtain gratification that he was not receiving in other spheres. For example, when he was younger, for a long time he had wanted to have a car and had not been able to afford it. "It was like having a car was a kind of gratification. I thought maybe my eating was trying to get the gratification that I wanted from having a car. So I thought that if I bought a car I might be able to lose weight. In those days I wanted a car so badly *that I could taste it.* But of course when I got the car, it didn't help.

"All these things are just rationalizations for why I really eat. They're excuses . . . They fool me. It's like a battle between me as an individual and my appetite. I try tricks and sometimes I can fool my appetite, and then it turns right around and tricks me."

Much of what Mr. Cohen told me in those early days was formulated in terms of "victories" and "defeats," or of instances of when "I was good" or "I was bad." The "victories," when he was "good," invariably involved instances of resisting the temptation to eat, reminiscences about experiences on diets, accounts of amounts of weight, often very large, that he had lost during earlier attempts at dieting. Conversely, "defeats" and "being bad" were instances of succumbing to the temptation to eat, of breaking a diet, of going to some absurd length to "prevent anyone from witnessing the shameful act I was just about to perform.

"Just yesterday, for example, I did a thing that makes no sense at all. I knew my wife had left something to eat in a closet in the kitchen. I kept thinking about it all the time, couldn't get it out of my mind. Then when she went to take a bath, I slipped in and stole it and ate it. Then I suddenly realized that naturally she would notice that it was gone when she looked in the closet again. So all of my elaborate precautions to avoid being discovered were pointless. Why do I do things like that?"

I shrugged my shoulders, "What kind of food was it?"

He frowned. "You know, I can't remember.

"I am a sleepwalker, too, you know," he volunteered. "My wife says that I do it every night sometimes. Usually I'm terribly angry. I'm shouting about somebody and I'm mad at them. It's always a man, 'George' or 'Dick' or something like that. I don't know who. And I eat then too. My wife says that I act in a very rational way. I get up, go to the icebox, get out food and eat it. And I have absolutely no memory of it the next morning. What do you think of that, Doc?"

Even his dreams reflected his concern with eating. "In this one dream this neighbor lady of ours was at dinner with my wife and me, and we were all eating roast stuffed veal. That's one of my favorite foods. Then, later, I was walking on the Lower East Side and I was gnawing a large, greasy piece of veal I had picked out of a garbage can. People were standing there watching me make a spectacle of myself, and I felt terribly ashamed of how I must look. But there wasn't anything I could do about it. Then that same night I had another dream. My fingernails were bitten to the quick. They were bleeding and I was sucking the blood. I felt miserable."

I suggested that we try to learn more about the circumstances under which his over-eating took place. It was clear that although he often ate at night, he was not suffering from the night-eating pattern. But perhaps his over-eating followed some pattern. I suggested that he pay particular attention to the times when he over-ate most heavily, and that we try to see if we could find any pattern in these occasions.

He applied himself diligently to the task, but at first without success. He seemed to eat in a chaotic manner throughout the day. Almost any kind of frustration, or achievement, could trigger his eating. Nevertheless, he began to feel better, the intense pressure to eat slackened, and he began to lose weight. It was under these circumstances, six weeks after he entered treatment, that he described the events which led me to recognize a second eating pattern.

The appointment began with a long pause. Then Mr. Cohen said, "I suppose you noticed the weight gain."

I nodded. His weight, which had fallen to 265 pounds in the previous six weeks, was again 272 pounds.

He started to talk two or three times, but could not. He looked up at the ceiling and then towards the door in an agony of embarrassment. Finally, he took a deep breath and said, "Well, I have to begin some time."

He began to talk about New Year's Day, two days before. He had told his wife that he was going down town to his chess club. While on the highway he began to think of going over to Newark to see a burlesque show. "So I did it. Just like that. As soon as the idea came into my mind I just went ahead and went over to Minsky's . . . Naturally I couldn't tell my wife about it . . . I hadn't seen a burlesque show in years. It was like when I was young."

Puzzled, I asked about his eating.

"No problem with eating. I kept it under 1000 calories," he said.

"Well, then, the weight . . . ?" I asked.

"That was the next day. I got my check cashed. I usually eat to celebrate the occasion. I don't have any idea why. So I knew it might happen. On the way to the bank I steeled myself. I kept reminding myself of the treatment and about my New Year's resolution about dieting and about having to face you and the scales."

He continued, slowing down to a less frantic pace. "Then I got the check cashed. And I kept out a hundred dollars. And everything just seemed to go blank. I don't know what happened. All of my good intentions just seemed to fade away. They just didn't seem to mean anything any more. I just said, 'What the hell,' and I started eating, and what I did then was an absolute sin."

He detailed what he had eaten. It was a tremendous amount and he had gained eight pounds during that one day. He had started in a grocery store, where he had bought a cake, pieces of pie and cookies, and he told of driving through the heavy midtown traffic with one hand, while pulling food out of the bag and eating it with the other.

After consuming all his grocery purchases as rapidly as possible, he had set out on a furtive round of the local restaurants, staying only a short time in each and eating only a small amount. Constantly in dread of discovery, he was not at all sure what "sin" he felt he was committing. He only knew that it wasn't pleasurable. "I didn't enjoy it at all. It just happened. It's like part of me blacked out, just wasn't there any more. And when that happened there was nothing there except the food and me—all alone."

Finally, he went into a delicatessen, bought another twenty dollars worth of food and drove home, eating all the way, "until my gut ached from all that I had eaten.

"My wife knew what I was doing, but she knows enough not to make an issue of it. Only later, in the evening, she seemed kind of wistful and asked me, 'When are you going to see Dr. Stunkard again?' "

Mr. Cohen sat looking ahead, a deep frown wrinkling his forehead. "And that's the whole truth, your honor."

I asked him how he felt, and he replied. "I feel some relief from telling you all this. I don't know why. Maybe it was like when I was seeing my analyst. I remember telling him about an eating binge. I had been walking down the street with nothing at all on my mind and looked across and saw a grocery store. The next thing I knew I was in the store

buying food. It was uncanny. It frightened me, not remembering how I had gotten there. But once I got started, there
wasn't a thing I could do about it. I remember that time
I spent $25 on groceries, and I had them in a big basket
and I hired a taxi and was riding all over New York eating
up a storm, eating away until my gut ached." He began to
laugh as he told of this earlier "binge," and he went on roaring
with laughter as he told of the long taxi ride which ended
at his home with a half-empty basket of food.

The memory of that earlier "binge," and of discussing
it with his analyst, persisted. "I had a very significant dream
that time," he said, and went on to describe quite vividly
a dream which must have occurred at least four years before.

"I was in a subway, on the Broadway-Seventh Avenue
line just after it comes out of the ground. The car was filled
with nude girls who were skipping rope. I wanted them to
let me in on the fun, but they excluded me. I was very sad
when I woke up."

Mr. Cohen said that he remembered that when he had
awakened from this dream he felt that it had been very
significant, and could hardly wait to tell his analyst. "It was
like he would be able to tell me what my problem was, and
then everything would be solved. Sort of like magic. And my
analyst was great. He told me, 'That's easy. That dream is
about *Man on a Tightrope.*' That was a book I had just read
and we had been talking about. It was about a man who
was unfaithful to his wife."

I asked what the analyst had meant, and Mr. Cohen
said, "I don't know except that I was having trouble with
my wife at that time. My analyst never said much, but that
was what he was talking about, about the trouble with my
wife. It reminded me of a quotation from Oscar Wilde: 'Most
men would be unfaithful to their wives if they weren't so
lazy.' That's the way I am. I've never been unfaithful, but
I would be, without any compunction, if the opportunity arose.
But I won't go looking."

Mr. Cohen's comments kept coming back towards his
wife. I thought of his trip to the burlesque show the day before

the binge, how he had introduced the topic of his weight gain by talking about that trip, and how he had taken it for granted that he could not tell his wife about it. I suggested that he tell me more about what had happened that day.

Mr. Cohen said that he wasn't at all sure how this was related to his eating, but he would be glad to talk about it. "There was a party at the neighbors' and everyone had been talking about pornography. I'm interested in pornography, and I was very interested when they talked about going to a burlesque show. But my wife didn't like it at all. She said that she thought it was all pretty disgusting. So I found myself saying the same thing too, that it was pretty disgusting. But I really would have liked to go, and if my wife had said she wanted to, I would have. Then some of the neighbors invited some of the people who had been at the party to see pornographic movies they had rented, and they didn't ask me. I felt terribly left out. I felt that if I hadn't talked like such a prude at the party they would have asked me to see the pornographic movies. That just stuck in my mind. That was what I was thinking about when I decided to go over to Minsky's. I don't know why it was so important to me."

This account of Mr. Cohen's marked a turning point in my understanding. Until then I had been overwhelmed, as had he, by what seemed a chaotic, patternless quality to his over-eating. But his talk of "an eating binge" had caught my attention. Although these binges might occur at night, their form was clearly quite different from the night-eating pattern. Here, it seemed, was a distinctive behavior; it might be possible to characterize it as fully as the night-eating pattern. Eagerly I set about this task, and, caught up by my enthusiasm, Mr. Cohen also threw himself into it.

First, what did it feel like when he was over-eating?

"There are two things I notice when I am eating like that. First of all, I just love the feeling of swallowing. I have my mouth full of food and I'm gulping it down, hardly even bothering to chew it, just stuffing it down. Then there's the feeling in my stomach, a full feeling, a very full feeling. It gets so full that it's painful, and I think that that's one of the things I'm looking for in a binge—eating so damned much that my gut aches. When that happens, then I can usually call off the binge, and a damned good thing, too. I might split my stomach wide open with all that I eat.

"Then, often I'll be drinking during a binge. I'll have a craving for spicy foods and this will make me thirsty, and so I'll drink beer. I might polish off six or eight bottles of beer just to keep me going, and then I'll want more food."

And how did he feel during these binges?

"Well," he began slowly, "I wonder. Sometimes I think maybe it's fun to be eating that way. But I don't know. I don't think it's fun. I usually feel pretty bad while I'm eating. I don't feel I'm in control any more. It's like I'm being driven to it."

And how did he feel after the binge? What was it like then?

"Well, there's this ache in my gut, and sometimes it gets pretty bad. It used to get bad enough that I would make myself vomit, to get all that stuff out of there. I'd forgotten about that. I used to do it quite a lot before my analysis, but I haven't done it at all since then. I guess the analysis cured me of it. But I remember now how I would make myself vomit, and then go back and start eating all over again."

"And what then?" I asked.

"I'd just feel like hell. I'd feel that I should be punished for my sins." He smiled in embarrassment. "There should be some retribution for the shameful act that I had performed."

I don't remember Mr. Cohen ever saying that he felt like a murderer in the aftermath of an eating binge, but I was to hear others talk this way. When I commented about the images he used to describe himself after a binge, saying that he seemed to feel like a criminal, he replied, as if it were the most obvious thing in the world, "of course."

As I thought about this exaggerated feeling of guilt, it occurred to me that I didn't remember Mr. Cohen ever having expressed guilt about anything else in his life. Had he felt so guilty about things other than eating? The answer was "no."

I briefly entertained the notion that his strong sense of guilt might have prevented any kind of activity that would make him feel guilty. But this supposition seemed unlikely on the face of it. He was an unusually energetic man, and I already knew that his Rabelaisian tastes extended far beyond eating. Indeed, as treatment continued, and as he came to trust me, he unfolded tales of activities that were antisocial, sometimes criminal. Far from being guilt-ridden, he experienced no qualms about any of them.

Even in early childhood he had stolen money from the cash register of his parents' store. There was a long history of cheating on his income tax and of passing bad checks. He consistently stole books from the library and pilfered small items from drugstores. His reckless driving resulted in a stream of traffic violations.

"I'm really a very amoral person," he observed. "But I don't feel guilty about anything except eating. Last term I stole a purse from one of the teachers at my school and made off with the $40 in it. She had left it in my office and forgotten it. At first I wasn't planning to steal it. I just hid it, planning to play a joke on her. But then later she told me she thought someone had taken it from her office. I realized she would never suspect me. So I took the money out and then took the purse home and burned it."

There was just one time that I remember Mr. Cohen saying he felt guilty over stealing. He described an episode at the house of a boy he was tutoring, while he was alone in the living room waiting for the boy to appear. "There was a big box of candy there and I started to eat it. I got a piece of sticky candy, and while I was chewing it, a filling came out. It was just terrible. 'Now I'll have to have a big dental job and it's going to cost me a lot of money.' " His shoulders slumped. He looked contrite. And when he spoke it was in a low, despairing tone, *"Things like that could ruin me."*

The guilt after an eating binge had one striking consequence. It often drove Mr. Cohen to diet. Many things could start him dieting—it might be something as trivial as having gotten through the day with little food. But the diets that followed binges had a special desperate quality to them. This was true of the first diet he undertook after he started treatment. It was about four months after he first came to see me, and followed the trip to Minsky's burlesque and his subsequent binge.

He began the diet with a terrible urgency. "I am an extremist. I just have to get on a strict diet and get this weight off, come hell or high water." As had often happened with such guilt-inspired diets, he ate very little and lost weight rapidly. He was soon commenting, "Once I really get into a diet it gets easier, and I find it less and less difficult to avoid food." Everything seemed to favor the diet. "I think my stomach must have shrunk. This morning I went into the place where I usually have breakfast and ordered black coffee, and when they brought me the coffee, they also brought me a bagel, which I usually eat with it. I just looked at the bagel and it revolted me. It was actual physical revulsion," he explained proudly. "Now I know I am on my way."

Such success in dieting was accompanied this time, as on other, similar occasions, by exuberance and a heightened mood. "It's like magic . . . I can control myself with ease. There just isn't a struggle any more. Things that would have thrown me before now just slide off my back without a second thought. I've even got my wife convinced. You remember how she used to feel about my coming here? Well, now she says she *believes* in psychiatry.

"The funny thing is, Doctor, that even hunger pangs feel good. They are really pleasurable; they make me feel as if I'm accomplishing something."

But these accomplishments were not to last. Hyman Cohen himself noted the fatal flaw. "The trouble with being an extremist," he observed, "is that it works the other way too. If I don't diet perfectly, I just give up. I say 'Oh hell, what's the use?' And then everything goes to hell and I just eat or drink. I might drink four quarts of beer, or a fifth of whiskey, and eat until my gut aches."

A month after starting the diet, and 25 pounds lighter, Mr. Cohen failed to diet perfectly and promptly gave up. It was a sequence he had repeated 20 times before. This time, however, there was a difference which made a profound impression upon Mr. Cohen, and intrigued and puzzled me. He stopped biting his fingernails for the first time in his life, and he never started again.

The vividness with which this highly intelligent man described events taught me a great deal about the distinctive pattern he called, appropriately enough, an "eating binge." My later experience with other patients confirmed much of what Mr. Cohen had taught me about this kind of over-eating: the sudden, out-of-the-blue way it came on, its orgiastic quality, the feeling of loss of control, and the compulsion to eat until the stomach was full, even painful.

There was also a pattern to the after-effects. One of the more dramatic was self-induced vomiting, which often allowed the binge to continue. Binges were usually followed by awesome distress and expressions of the most bitter self-condemnation, usually focused on the eating itself, and rarely on inter-personal concerns. Finally, the binge and the later guilt were often followed by quixotically austere diets, usually of very short duration.

Together Mr. Cohen and I began to recognize these eating binges as discrete events, identifying when they occurred, how long they lasted, and what happened afterward. Now we turned to the next question. What started them?

It had been relatively easy to discover the characteristics and consequences of the binges themselves; it was much harder to find a pattern in what preceded them. But the search was important. For understanding the events that precipitate eating binges led, often quite directly, to understanding the major problems in a patient's life. And sometimes the solutions to these problems led to control of their obesity.

Trying to discover the cause of Mr. Cohen's eating binges seemed at first quite hopeless. Practically everything he did appeared to bring on a binge. He would binge whenever he cashed a check and had money in his hand, or whenever he went to the Household Finance Corporation and came out with a loan. He would binge to reward himself after he finished a hard job. He would binge to celebrate when he had signed up a new student for tutoring. He would binge when he felt "down in the dumps and didn't give a damn," or when he was feeling expansive, "like a Kwakiutl Indian giving a potlatch."

But gradually, as the binges became less frequent, Mr. Cohen learned to focus his attention more and more sharply upon the period preceding them. Slowly, over a period of many weeks, a pattern began to appear.

In retrospect, there had been clues as early as the third visit. Looking back at my notes for that hour, I saw a remark that had struck me at the time. In describing his over-eating, Mr. Cohen had said, "There is this curious feeling, sometimes, that I'm getting even with someone. It's a vague feeling and it sounds queer to me. I don't know who I'm angry at, or why."

After a pause he had gone on to say that he got angry at his mother when she seemed to disapprove of his eating. "And then I ate as if I meant to spite her."

The second clue came from the binge after his visit to Minsky's burlesque; this was the first time he had referred to problems with his wife. He had made the casual comment that "naturally" he couldn't tell her about the burlesque show. And he went on to talk about his dream years before of nude girls dancing in the subway, and how he associated the dream with marital troubles. Finally, and most importantly, he spoke of his feelings about having been left out of the pornographic picture show because of his prudish remarks which had followed his wife's lead.

As we discussed these events over the next few weeks, it became apparent that not only had Hyman Cohen felt left out, he had felt intense resentment. Most of all he had been distressed at his own passivity in having followed his wife's lead, and in having expressed sentiments about the pornography that were almost the opposite of those he really felt.

We gradually learned that anger played a critical role in his binges; and, as treatment continued, he became more aware of this anger. One incident was particularly instructive.

He had been given the responsibility of disciplining a fourteen year-old boy who had a record of truancy. The boy had defied Mr. Cohen, who suddenly found himself slapping him. "I don't know how it happened. I didn't have the vaguest thought of doing anything like that. But when I saw that little monster sneering at me, I guess I just lost control. I didn't mean to hit him. I just wanted to overawe him. But when he looked so defiant, I just got furious." Then, with a casualness which belied the significance of his remark, he said, "If I hadn't hit that boy, I know I would have gone out and had a binge."

The next week, by contrast, he got angry on two occasions and had not been able to do anything about the anger. He arrived for his appointment three pounds heavier.

By the time Mr. Cohen was able to embark upon a serious, sustained diet, his relationship with his wife had begun to deteriorate. This unfortunate development had one favorable consequence: it greatly facilitated the identification of events that precipitated eating binges. His binges occurred when he had been infuriated by his wife. This fury, however, did not always result in an eating binge. At times it led to physical violence—and twice caused injuries to his wife serious enough to require medical attention. Never after such violence did he have an eating binge.

By the second year of treatment, we could generalize further about the anger which precipitated binges: they usually followed a period during which he had not been able to respond effectively to the person who had angered him. Again and again we recognized situations like that of the party, when his wife had denounced pornography, and when, helpless and passive, he had found himself "selling out" and complying with another's wishes. Later, if he found that these wishes were not in his own best interest, he would feel powerless and betrayed. Mounting anger would set the stage for a binge.

The circumstances that had surrounded his first binges, at the age of 19 or 20, supported the idea that helplessness and passivity in response to threats to his integrity had regularly led to anger and binges. During college he had spent much of his spare time working in his parents' bakery and later in a delicatessen. The family had been very poor, and he had felt humiliated by the poverty and "degraded" by having to wear an apron in the bakery, "like a shopkeeper, deferring to the wishes of others."

One event in particular stuck in his mind. When he had been working in the delicatessen, an Irish Catholic youth had been dissatisfied with a frankfurter Mr. Cohen had served him. Voicing his scorn, he threw it at Mr. Cohen, mustard and all, splattering his clean clothes. "I remember thinking at the time, 'Here I am, aspiring to a professional career and having to cater to these crumbs and be subservient to them. I don't belong here. I am a displaced aristocrat, a member of the intellectual elite. And yet here I am, having to eat their shit . . .' "

Instead, he had eaten cakes and cookies. In those days, when his eating binges had had their start, Mr. Cohen ate what was at hand. In the delicatessen, a cake, possibly two, had served as a starter, followed by cookies, crackers, "anything at all," all washed down with a quart of milk.

The detail of Hyman Cohen's eating pattern, and the larger symptomatic picture into which it fell, formed the basis of my lecture at the psychiatric hospital. In it I described the night-eating pattern and contrasted it with the binge-eating pattern so well-exemplified by Hyman Cohen.

Afterwards, over coffee, the informal discussion became quite animated. "I don't get it," a tall dark young staff member remarked. "A friend of yours, a layman, refers a patient to you and tells you he is a compulsive eater. You treat him for two years and you end up with the conclusion that he is a compulsive eater. What's the big deal?" On that note, we embarked on the kind of discussion which had become very familiar.

Yes, it did appear that Mr. Cohen was a compulsive eater. But that was not the point I was trying to make. I was attempting to describe particular kinds of behavior so discrete and clearly defined that everyone could agree upon them. And I was hoping to use these descriptions of eating behavior to classify different kinds of human obesity.

"But that's nothing but descriptive psychiatry!", the tall, dark man exclaimed incredulously.

That comment usually ended discussions, for "descriptive psychiatry" was the antithesis of the "dynamic psychiatry," derived from psychoanalysis, which at that time dominated American psychiatry. "Dynamic psychiatry" had a positive aura about it. "Descriptive psychiatry" implied shallowness and superficiality, not getting to the root of problems, ineffective treatment.

I mulled over the choices for a time, and then agreed. Yes, it was descriptive psychiatry; but perhaps we needed some descriptive psychiatry. Dynamic psychiatry had not proved very helpful in advancing our understanding of human obesity.

The rather diffuse concept of compulsive eating provided a good example. By contrast, the notion of binge-eating is quite definite. While it is fairly easy to decide whether a person is a binge-eater, it may be very difficult to decide whether he is a compulsive eater. On the simplest level, "compulsion" is a descriptive term. It refers to a strong, often irresistible, inclination to carry out repetitive and often apparently meaningless acts. A well-known example is the hand-washing compulsion that drives people to wash their already clean hands 20, 30 and 40 times a day for no reason that they can recognize.

Some obese people do appear subject to strong inclinations to eat, and even over-eat, and Mr. Cohen was certainly a good example of this. But almost anyone who has gone without food for a time is strongly inclined to eat, and normal-weight people may be even more strongly inclined than many obese ones. When "compulsive eating" is defined in these older, descriptive terms, it accounts for the over-eating of no more than a small minority of obese people.

But compulsions can also be considered in terms of the psychic apparatus which is presumed to underlie them. According to this view, the origins of compulsions are found in the conflict between a drive and the defense mechanisms opposed to that drive. Under appropriate circumstances, the intensity of the conflict is decreased by isolating the psychic energy attached to the drive and displacing it onto some neutral topic. For example, the intensity of a hostile drive towards a husband may be decreased by displacing the energy which activates it onto a neutral act such as hand-washing. The conflict-ridden housewife thereby becomes less tense in the presence of her husband, but at the expense of repetitive, apparently meaningless, hand-washing.

This is the sort of compulsion which seemed to precipitate Mr. Cohen's eating binges, and understanding them appeared helpful in his treatment. But it had taken a great deal of hard work to reach this point. And it seemed unlikely that the diagnosis of compulsive eating could be made in anyone without a similarly arduous effort. If so, we are able to discover who is a compulsive eater only by a process so cumbersome that we will probably never be able to identify more than a few of them.

What are the implications of eating binges? What does this diagnosis tell us about the kind of person who binges and the hope of controlling his obesity? How many obese people are binge-eaters? It is clearly an uncommon disorder, and it is difficult for any one investigator to draw conclusions about it from the limited number of binge-eaters he is likely to encounter. I have carefully studied no more than nine or ten.

In the course of this work, I have been surprised to discover that binge-eating is not confined to obese people. It is even more commonly associated with anorexia nervosa, a rare disorder that afflicts primarily females, particularly adolescents, who voluntarily restrict their food intake so uncompromisingly that many become walking skeletons and some even die. As many as 50 per cent may eat in binges. In fact, the frightening experience of losing control and gorging on food seems to play a large part in the rigid restrictions these young women put upon their eating. Some say that they feel that the slightest freedom in eating would result in a total loss of control. And the diets they undertake with such drastic effect are often frighteningly austere, even bizarre, surpassing in intensity those of obese binge-eaters. It is perhaps not surprising that many of them have a morbid fear of becoming obese.

Fortunately, there is a paradox about binge-eating which offers some grounds for optimism regarding treatment. Binge-eaters usually have severe emotional disturbances, which are little helped by the emotional support of family, friends and physicians—or even by extensive weight reduction. Yet the results of treatment (of the few who have undergone prolonged psychotherapy) have been surprisingly good. The treatment has frequently been stormy and always prolonged. But a few binge-eaters have not only resolved their emotional difficulties, they have lost a great deal of weight in the process.

The binges themselves may even be an asset, for an understanding of the events which cause eating binges frequently leads directly to the major conflicts which disturb the patient.

six

Physical Activity

Hyman Cohen's story did not end with the study of binge-eating, nor was it ever confined to that inquiry. Over the 14 years that he was my patient, many concerns influenced his treatment. An important one was the extent of his physical activity.

The relationship between physical activity and obesity had long fascinated me. There was a great deal of folklore about how inactive—"lazy" is the usual term—obese people were. But it took Jean Mayer to give the belief scientific respectability. Observing obese girls at a summer camp he found that they were significantly less active than their non-obese counterparts. In fact, their inactivity was so marked that it could account for their obesity all by itself, without any over-eating.

Interesting as this was, Mayer's next finding was even more important. When he subjected normal rats to differing periods of exercise in a running wheel, he found that, under most circumstances, they were able to regulate their body weight with great precision. Beginning with one hour a day in the wheel and gradually increasing their exercise to as many as eight hours a day, he observed the following: with each increment in activity the rats increased their eating just enough to compensate for the extra calories they burned up. As a result body weight remained constant.

When the physical activity of the rats fell below one hour a day, however, there were astonishingly different results. Any decrease in physical activity led to an increase in food intake! Conversely, increasing the physical activity (while remaining below the critical limit of one hour) decreased their food intake.

The effects upon body weight were predictable. Decreasing physical activity and increasing food intake led to a rapid gain in weight. On the other hand those rats whose physical activity was increased (to no more than an hour a day), and whose appetites decreased, lost weight.

This was really a remarkable finding. Its unexpected, paradoxical quality, so characteristic of great discoveries, continues to intrigue me. I cannot help but feel that we have still not realized all of its implications, but some of them were clear (and profoundly important) from the beginning.

We already knew that the great increase in obesity in our affluent society had not resulted simply from the greater availability of food. Adequate amounts of food had been available for large segments of our population for many years. The widespread decrease in physical activity seemed a more likely cause, as one mechanical device after the other had taken over the tasks formerly carried out by human muscles.

But until Mayer's discovery it was not apparent how this decrease in physical activity had led to obesity. If people were regulating their body weight correctly, the decrease in physical activity should have been accompanied by an equivalent decrease in the amount they ate. Evidently this wasn't happening. But why?

We can assume that the answer lies in our technological advances. In the United States of many years ago, as in many underdeveloped areas today, the activity level of most people was probably high enough to cause a more or less automatic regulation of their food intake (like Mayer's rats who ran more than one hour a day). With greater technological development, however, our physical activity may have fallen to whatever is the human equivalent of the rats' running less than one hour a day. And like the sedentary rats, our decreased physical activity may actually be increasing our eating.

If these assumptions are even approximately correct, they are bright with promise for the control of obesity. They suggest that an increase in physical activity may help to control obesity, not just because of the extra calories burned up, but more importantly, by moving obese people back to the level where food intake is more instinctively related to physical activity.

As striking as these findings were, it was well over a year after learning of them before I started to work on the topic. Much as I had wanted to earlier, I had no idea of where to begin. Then one day on impulse I dropped into an instrument store whose window display had long intrigued me. I had always wanted an excuse to buy one of the shiny, fascinating and overpriced instruments which were so artfully displayed. Behind a pocket-watch sized instrument was the sign: "Pedometer. Find out how far you walk. Wear it on the golf course or at work. Amaze your family and friends." Without a moment's hesitation I bought one; and since that first purchase, I have regularly used pedometers, measuring my own activity daily for 3 years, and my patients for even longer.

In the initial study of physical activity, I was joined by a medical student. Ronald Dorris had impressed me by the

seriousness and skill with which he approached the treatment
of patients, and I was pleased that he was interested in learning
more about obesity. A handsome, modest young man, quiet
and enormously capable, he supported my probably exaggerated regard for Harvard graduates. And he seemed quite
agreeable to the idea of trying out pedometers on obese people.
By comparing the distance which each of them walked each
day with that of a non-obese person, we expected to be able
to find out if the obese people were indeed less active—and
if so, how much less active. Dorris enthusiastically responded
to this suggestion. In fact, he gave it an elegant twist.

While we were planning the study, Dorris suggested that
it might be interesting to investigate the attitudes toward
physical activity, as well as the physical activity itself. I agreed,
and then learned that he knew a great deal about the topic.
While still an undergraduate he had helped to develop a
sentence-completion test which he had used to study attitudes,
and particularly how conscious people were of their attitudes.
We discussed what kinds of attitudes towards activity we might
expect to find, and then Dorris prepared a sentence-completion test embodying these ideas. It consisted of 15 paired,
open-ended sentence fragments, half of which used the first
person pronoun and half of which used the third person
pronoun.

From the first we suspected that depression might play
a part in attitudes towards activity, and Dorris prepared the
beginning of sentences to test this idea. "When I am blue,
I . . ." explored the subjects' conscious appraisal of what they
would do when depressed. The same inquiry was worded in
the third person: "When she's down in the dumps, she . . ."
Dorris had found that, through this third-person device he
could sometimes uncover attitudes which subjects would be
too self-conscious to admit in the first person.

We confined the study to obese women, who outnum-
bered men by 9 to 1 in the hospital clinics. Dorris reviewed
the records of these patients to exclude any who had some
physical disability other than obesity, which might affect their
physical activity. We were surprised at how few there were.

The overwhelming proportion of obese people who sought medical attention had no associated physical disabilities.

When we compared the activity of those obese women with that of a control group of matched, non-obese women, we found a striking difference. The obese women were far less active than the non-obese women. Whereas the latter walked 4.5 miles a day, the obese women walked no more than 1.5.

The sentence-completion test showed differences which were almost as marked. Sentences probing the women's response to depression were particularly impressive. Every one of the obese women reported a passive acceptance of a depressed mood. Typical responses were: "When I am blue, I *just cry,*" and "When she is down in the dumps, she *just sulks.*" The non-obese women, on the other hand, frequently gave responses which indicated that they were struggling against feelings of despondency. Typical ones were: "When I am blue, I *clean house,*" and "When she is down in the dumps, she *counts her blessings.*"

We had also attempted to assess the subjects' attitudes toward boredom, a complaint which I had heard all too often from obese patients. Again the results indicated more passive responses on the part of the obese women: "When I am not interested, I *get depressed,*" and "When she's bored, she *often shows it.*" Although some of the non-obese women gave similar responses, the majority replied in a more active vein: "When I am not interested, I *read,*" and "When she's bored, she *irons clothes.*"

Social interaction is a major stimulus to physical activity, and we therefore tried to assess the subjects' attitudes toward it. Again we found significant differences between the two groups. The obese women usually gave responses suggesting far less capacity to develop easy relationships with other people: "Working with people makes me feel *no different than working alone,*" and "The others in the office make her feel *isolated.*" The non-obese women, on the other hand, evidenced a remarkable degree of confidence in their ability to form good social relations. Typical responses were: "Working with people makes me feel *just perfect,*" and "The others in the office make her feel *welcome.*"

These clear-cut results elated us. This was the first study to actually measure the physical activity of obese people, and it showed clearly the part played by lessened physical activity. Furthermore, the correlation between activity and attitudes suggested that any attempt to increase physical activity was going to have to deal with the self-defeating attitudes of the obese. Prominent among these attitudes were those indicating depression. Did depression lie behind the inactivity of obese people? One way of approaching the problem was to measure their levels of physical activity over a period of time and see if these related to the presence and intensity of their depression.

Once again I turned to my patients. Would they be willing to wear a pedometer and keep a record of their physical activity? Everyone whom I asked agreed, and I immediately began to keep daily records of their physical activity.

This was where Hyman Cohen proved particularly helpful. From our second meeting on, he had repeatedly asked if he could take part in some kind of research. For a time I had demurred, trying to understand his reasons. But I finally decided that his self-esteem would be buoyed by viewing himself as a collaborator in medical research. And I was coming to the conclusion that his treatment was going to be a long one, allowing plenty of time to work out any complications engendered by the dual relationship.

During the first weeks of treatment, Mr. Cohen walked no more than 2.0 miles a day. As he explained it, "You have no idea how lazy I am, Doc. I've got a card catalogue in my office and when I'm working on it lots of times I'll send for a student messenger to get the cards rather than walk across the room . . . Why I'll take the car if I've only got three blocks to go, even if I have to park so far away from where I am going that I'll have to walk more than three blocks to get there. I'm that lazy."

We spent a good deal of time talking about his inactivity, and he attributed much of it to his sweating. "You see, I sweat so easily, Doc, especially when I exercise, and all that sweat just makes me feel uncomfortable. It chafes my skin too, especially around the crotch, and I would do anything rather than sweat."

Very soon after Mr. Cohen began to keep a record of his physical activity, there occurred the significant events surrounding his trip to the burlesque show and the explosive eating binge which had followed. The pedometer measurements during this brief period told a striking story: During the nine days before the fateful party at which he supported his wife's condemnation of pornography, Mr. Cohen had walked an average of 2.1 miles a day. For the following three days he kept no record of his activity. Then followed six days of depression with an average of 0.5 mile a day. On the day of the eating binge his activity returned to its former level; and during the next nine days, with the lifting of the depression, he again walked an average of 2.1 miles a day.

Here was a very close association between a severely depressed mood (superimposed on a more chronic depression) and a marked reduction in physical activity. Not being invited to watch the pornographic movies had been a devastating blow on three counts. First, Mr. Cohen was a sexually very active man with a strong fascination for all aspects of the topic. He would have liked nothing better than to watch the pornographic movies. Second, he had at least the usual sensitivity to rejection, and he felt doubly rejected because the friends who had invited him to a conventional party had excluded him from a gathering in which he would have had a far greater interest. Third, and most important, was his betrayal of himself. He was well aware of his intense curiosity about sex. His prudish protestations, in imitation of his wife's, had been a shameless sell-out.

It was only later in treatment that I began to understand this passivity toward his wife and his inability to acknowledge what seemed to be strong evidence of hostility toward her. Some further description of Hyman Cohen and his past may help explain the reasons.

Hyman Cohen was the older of two sons born in New York to a Jewish immigrant couple from Eastern Europe. He maintained that he had no memories before the age of eight,

and at no time during our long association did I find any
evidence to contradict this unusual assertion. So I was unable
to ascertain early childhood influences upon his later behavior.
But even earlier influences, genetic ones, seemed to play a
role.

His father was very obese and suffered from a manic
depressive psychosis which hospitalized him for the last 30
years of his life. His mother was also obese, and the obesity
of the two made it unlikely that he would escape the condition.
He did escape the mental deterioration which afflicted his
father and was never hospitalized. But throughout his life
he showed milder manic depressive features: a strong tendency
to elation or, less frequently, depression; the ability to deny
undeniable problems; and a lack of sensitivity (or psycho-
logical-mindedness).

Mr. Cohen's earliest memory was when his father had
left home. He remembered his mother telling him about it
and recalled his mixed feelings—sadness at his father's leaving,
but pride at what his mother told him his father was going
to do. She apparently had controlled her disappointment and
told her baseball-loving son that his father had moved west
to manage the Detroit Tigers. He learned much later that
his father had been fired from his job after a fight with his
boss, and had left town to work as a traveling salesman.

The other memories were bitter ones. There was the time
when his father could not answer a neighbor who asked what
grade his son was in. On another occasion, when he had
declined his father's invitation to go to a boxing match, his
father ferociously scolded him "for not being a red-blooded
American boy."

But the bitterest disappointment occurred when he was
17 years old. Hyman Cohen had undergone an appendectomy
and was waiting in the hospital, when he was surprised by
the appearance of his father, whom he had thought was out
of town. His father bundled him into the car to drive him
home, and when they arrived, let him out of the car, and
drove on to park it. When Mr. Cohen went to the front door,
he found himself too weak to open it, and he waited for his
father to return and open it for him. But his father never

came, and he finally sat down in front of the house and cried. "I felt helpless and completely neglected by my father. It was just the worst time in my life. And that's what started my weight problem. I just decided that I would eat and eat until I had built my strength up. And of course I just didn't stop."

Actually Mr. Cohen had been overweight most of his life, but it became more severe after this incident; and it was this incident which he came to view as a specific cause of his obesity.

"After that, Dad appeared only very briefly, and not very often. I remember he once appeared in a tremendous old green Lincoln touring car with a Negro chauffeur. He was walking around the neighborhood telling people about the big business deals he was making and borrowing money from them. This was very embarrassing to my mother and me, and the store wasn't doing very well either."

Mr. Cohen was 19 the last time his father appeared. "Sometimes he would be very dapper and well-dressed. But this time he wasn't. He looked terrible. He was dirty and had a beard, and a dead cigar butt in his mouth that he kept chewing on. He wasn't making much sense, and then he tried to assault Mother sexually. I had to threaten him with a baseball bat to get him to let her alone. We had to commit him then, and I don't think this was the first time. But he never got out of the hospital after that."

Mr. Cohen's memories of his mother were less unreservedly negative. They weren't really joyful memories either—I sometimes thought of them as bitter-sweet. "I guess the happiest memories of my life were of times with Mother. I must have been about 13, I can't remember exactly, and my mother had a job in a candy store out in Throgg's Neck. The high point of my week was going out there by trolley on Saturday night and helping her put together the Sunday papers and then coming back with her on the trolley after midnight on Sunday."

Mr. Cohen often told me about these Saturday nights, and he kept coming back to them. "I can fix one date around that time very accurately, the closing of the banks in March of 1933. I have a clear recollection of my parents standing in line for many hours trying to withdraw their account."

Throughout Mr. Cohen's youth financial difficulties plagued the family, and his mother never escaped from the frightened, penurious world of those days. She was always worrying about money. Many years later when Mr. Cohen bought his first car, his mother was terribly upset and begged him again and again to be more careful with his money.

After one of the occasions when his father lost his job, there was a large family meeting to plot the proper course for his parents. It was decided that they should run a bakery, and his mother's family bought it for them. "That was a confused and uncomfortable period. It must have been about that time that Dad left home and had some sort of a job as a traveling salesman. We moved in with some of my mother's family in very crowded conditions up in the Bronx.

"Then I can remember another family conference. It was very tense. My uncle Sam threatened to beat Dad up if he didn't do better. I remember he said he'd beat the be-Jesus out of him. Then they loaned my mother $1700 to buy the bakery. We kept living with her sisters and her mother all of this time, and it was terribly hard work. We'd open up at six in the morning and stay open till midnight. There wasn't any family life at all. And that went on for seven years."

Mr. Cohen's account of a childhood lived in close relationship to food stores is a very common one among obese men. It has seemed to me that a majority of them have either been raised by a family involved with a food business, or have had a food-related occupation themselves, or both. Of course this was not so unusual in New York, from which most of my patients originally came, and where there is such a profusion of small confectionary shops. These are often run by Jews, and obesity in Jewish men and boys is not unusual. For women the association between food occupations and obesity is not nearly so close. One can speculate that this is because the average woman has so much more to do with food in the course of her personal daily routine.

Despite all the turmoil of these years, Mr. Cohen graduated from high school and started college. But financial pressures soon forced him to cut down to one course at college in order to help his mother with the bakery. He was pursuing this dual career at the age of 19 when his father had returned home for the last time. Perhaps his father's hospitalization ended any hope of improvement in the family finances. In any event, his mother sold the bakery to pay for her son to attend college full time. She got a job working in a sister's delicatessen (and was still working there during the time I treated her son).

Such devotion on the part of his mother might have repaired Mr. Cohen's loss of his father. But the days with Mother were not all bliss—and not simply because of her financial insecurities. When Mr. Cohen was 8 years old, the year that his father had first left home, his mother had had a second son. And this son received most of what his mother liked to call her "love." From Hyman she had demanded companionship and performance; he had been flattered, and had complied. From his brother she demanded nothing except the chance to give. Or, as Hyman Cohen's wife was later to remark in her acid manner, "If you were her husband, your brother was her lover."

Mr. Cohen grew up with an intense jealousy of this spoiled young darling and a lifelong impairment of his ability to relate to younger men and boys. His experience with his father had left him with a hopeless yearning and a real despair of ever being able to trust an older man. Clearly, these emotions underlay his identification with his psychiatrist and his intense dependence upon him.

But basically Mr. Cohen looked to women for his security, and his search was desperate, unrelenting and compulsive. Despite his puritanical background and its financial strictures, he had begun to make the rounds of prostitutes long before he had emerged from adolescence. And graduation from college and entry into wartime military service had signaled the onset of almost frantic sexual activity. Until the age of 23 all of this activity was with prostitutes.

Then, one day when he was on furlough, forlorn and homesick, he met a "nice girl" and she took him to bed. "I married her three weeks later, out of gratitude. What else

could I do?" In response to my raised eyebrows, he continued,
"It was the first time I had ever had sex without having to
pay for it. I just felt so grateful to her that I didn't know
what to do. The least I could do was marry her."

Mr. Cohen's attitude toward his wife had this intense,
all-or-nothing quality. His relationship with her was for many
years one of unqualified awe. The first time he ever mentioned
her to me he said, "When I diet she praises me, and that
makes me feel like a good boy."

The bliss of the marriage cooled when his wife proposed
that they have a child, and things went downhill as the
proposal became a demand. For five years he put her off,
and her demands mounted. Finally, when Mr. Cohen was
28 years old, his wife played her trump card. Unless they
had a child, she would leave him.

"It was just awful. I couldn't live without her and yet
I couldn't stand the idea of being a father, I just wasn't ready
to be a father, and she forced me into it." For a time after
the birth of their son, Mr. Cohen had left his wife, but
he had crept back to her within a few weeks, contrite and
unhappy.

Over the years they had settled into an equilibrium of
unhappy mutual dependency. Only as we began to examine
the marriage in the course of treatment did he realize just
how unhappy they were.

The marriage never really survived the birth of their
son, Walter. Mr. Cohen was never able to shake the deep
conviction that his wife preferred Walter to him, and would
have left him had it not been for his siring her child. He
felt insecure, apprehensive, depressed. He felt betrayed at
having to be a father, and constantly avoided his son. And
he treated his wife as the betrayer, at times passively complaining to her, at others actively shouting and even hitting
her—all the while ridiculing her increasingly neurotic behavior. His wife, in turn, found that a child did not bring relief
from her intense suffering. Now she had to cope with her
baby alone, with no help from her increasingly estranged
husband. Adventurous and highly intelligent as a young

woman, she found herself restricted to a narrow round of household chores, which she carried out with mounting desperation.

It had struck me during Mr. Cohen's first mention of his wife, when he was describing their happy marriage, that he had laughed as he told me about how he frequently tried to choke her during his sleep. He similarly told me cheerful accounts of her "little rituals." One was to say "God keep Hyman safe," ten times before going to sleep—five times if they had had intercourse—and of her panic if he prevented enactment of the ritual.

It seemed as though that was the first time he had ever thought about the meaning of his wife's waxing the floors every day and her refusal to permit either shoes or bare feet on them; only slippers would protect the shiny luster of the floors she polished so religiously, and she would go into fits of screaming if her son walked on them in his bare feet. Mr. Cohen had long since given up hope of any such freedom.

He had never related the events in his daily life to the fluctuations in his weight, and it was difficult to reconstruct the relationships at this late date. After the experience of his father's abandonment following his appendectomy at age 17, Mr. Cohen's eating had soon brought his weight to 220 pounds. And there it remained through the military service which followed college. After he was released, at the age of 25, it had risen to nearly the 272 pounds which he weighed when he came to see me at the age of 37. This increase had been punctuated by frequent diets. And it was apparently the failure of one of these, and the consequent rapid increase in weight, which had caused him to seek treatment. He was depressed, over-eating and under-active—averaging only two miles a day.

By the time Hyman Cohen had finished telling me about his life, it was easy to understand his compliance with his wife's distaste for the pornographic movies, and his inability to acknowledge his strong hostility toward her. He was so terribly dependent upon her, and so uncertain of her support, that he did not dare to acknowledge even the slightest resentment. He could not be even appropriately self-assertive, for fear that such action might jeopardize that relationship. Locked in their unhappy embrace, the Cohens moved slowly towards tragedy.

The impact of treatment became apparent quite early. First there was a lessening in the intensity of Mr. Cohen's depression. There were also glimmerings of a reduced dependence upon his wife, and the first hints of criticism of her. The following months saw continuing improvement in his mood and a growing independence of his wife. His physical activity, however, increased only slightly, from 2 to 2.5 miles a day, and his weight remained at 270 pounds.

What led to this improvement? I attributed much of it to the strong positive transference which Mr. Cohen had developed towards me. It appeared that his dependent needs were being gratified, and he strongly identified with me, viewing us as fellow explorers in the trackless waste of obesity. I am inclined to believe that this kind of improvement will usually occur in the course of psychotherapy, provided the therapist does not interfere with it.

It was about this time, five months into Hyman Cohen's treatment, that I was offered an excellent position in the Department of Psychiatry at the University of Pennsylvania. Since the job promised new and exciting possibilities, I accepted; and with Dr. Wolff's blessings, I made plans to leave New York.

The move to Pennsylvania brought with it one of the most painful moments in a physician's life—parting from his patients. For some, termination of treatment was possible. For others, transfer to the care of another doctor seemed the wisest course. Hyman Cohen was among this second group. And one spring morning, I told him that I had discussed the situation with an excellent psychiatrist in New York, who would be happy to see him for treatment. I had developed a real affection for Hyman Cohen, and I told him how sorry I was that this development would end our relationship, one I had come to prize. Although I did not say it, I felt particularly unhappy at demonstrating to him once again the unreliability of older men, always leaving him when they were needed most.

Mr. Cohen's reaction to my departure was, in retrospect, understandable. He swallowed his disappointment and told me that if we only had two months left, he intended to make the most of it. He had no desire at all to see another doctor, and "I have decided here and now that I will get down to work and finish up this treatment in the two months that we have left."

It almost looked as if he were going to do just that. He came into the office the next week beaming, to announce that the preceding week had been the most successful since the start of treatment—in fact, one of the most successful he had ever known. He had embarked upon a reducing diet and had already lost six pounds, and he had begun to make a conscious effort to increase his physical activity.

These feelings of well-being continued and grew into what he called his "benzedrine syndrome." His energy became boundless, his need for sleep dropped to less than five hours a day, and everything took on a rosy glow. "It's like magic —your prediction has come true. Just by understanding my reactions, I can control my eating with no difficulty at all. It just isn't a struggle any more. Things which would have thrown me now slide off my back with no trouble. Even my wife says that now she believes in psychiatry. It really works. She has mentioned my nails growing out for the first time since she's known me, and how I can control my appetite, and she says that this is the best that she can remember."

He continued to diet, dropping from 270 to 250 pounds in six weeks. His activity shot up from 2.5 to 4.5 miles a day, an astonishing increase for him. He was clearly reacting to the threatened loss with his usual pattern of elation, and for a time I was worried about him. The circumstances seemed too similar to the first elated stage of a dieting depression.

Then Mr. Cohen took matters into his own hands. On our next-to-last appointment he began somewhat hesitantly

by saying that he had had a talk about my impending departure with the friend who referred him to me. Mr. Liebowitz
had suggested that he ask if he could come down to Philadelphia to see me. "So I'm putting the question to you, Doc."
I told him that I would be glad to see him in Philadelphia,
but pointed out some of the difficulties. He replied that since
school was already finished for the year there would be no
difficulty in his getting away from New York. We agreed to
try it out for the summer and then see how feasible it was
to continue after that.

This direct action towards a course which he desired,
and its favorable outcome, had a strong impact upon Mr.
Cohen. His self-confidence soared, and with it came an end
to the elation. His mood fell to a more appropriate level;
he began to sleep more regularly and for longer periods; and
his hyper-activity decreased. Pedometer measurements fell
from 4.5 miles a day to 3 miles a day, and they stayed at
this level for as long as he continued to make these measurements, a period of over two years. His weight also leveled
off at 250 pounds and continued at this level for several years.

In reviewing these long-term records of physical activity
and weight, I felt that they supported Mayer's discovery. Early
in treatment, when he was averaging 2 miles a day, Mr.
Cohen's weight had fluctuated around 270 pounds. Six months
later, when his physical activity had stabilized at 3 miles a
day, his weight also stabilized, at 250 pounds. Neither of these
measures showed appreciable long-term changes during the
tumultuous period which followed.

This period was ushered in, paradoxically, by Mr.
Cohen's steady progress in treatment. For this progress seemed
to disturb his wife, who became increasingly distraught and
apprehensive. The precarious equilibrium between them
eroded. As his increasing capacity for independence freed him
from his dependence on her, she became more and more
disturbed. A year of alcoholism was followed by another year
of increasingly bizarre behavior and periodic psychiatric hospitalizations. Three years after her husband had entered treatment, Mrs. Cohen committed suicide.

Mr. Cohen continued treatment with me over a period of 14 years, at first on a weekly basis, and later at infrequent intervals. And occasional letters keep me in touch with him to this day.

The years of turmoil were followed by years of loneliness. Gradually, however, Mr. Cohen came to accept his son and even to love him. Then he married a warm and loving woman and began the relationship which Mr. Cohen still feels is the best thing that ever happened to him. He qualified for the job as principal of his high school and for many years has coped well with the rigorous demands of this office. Throughout these years his weight has remained around 250 pounds.

The treatment of Hyman Cohen, which swept me into the tragedy and triumphs of his life, moved me deeply. It left me with a growing dissatisfaction with a therapy which could help an individual only at such a high cost to his family. And it raised serious doubts about the importance of mood-related changes in physical activity.

On the one hand, it was clear that depression was associated with decreases in physical activity. This combination had occurred so frequently and under so many different circumstances, that I no longer doubted that the two factors were linked. On the other hand, the comparative size of the changes in activity during depression was disappointingly small. Mr. Cohen walked 2 miles a day when he was depressed and 3 miles a day when he was not depressed. This 50 percent increase was highly significant from a statistical point of view; but in practical terms of increased calorie expenditure, it was far less impressive. It was only an extra twenty minutes of walking, no more than 200 Calories.

Some of the short-term periods of depression—such as the one which followed the disappointment about the pornographic movies—were associated with an even more severe reduction in physical activity. And the combination of depression and diminished physical activity probably made some contribution to his obesity. But the contrast between this contribution and others made it clear that other influences were far more important. The years of study and the collection of thousands of pedometer measurements provided a number of hunches as to what some of these influences were, and sufficient data to test them.

There seemed to be three sets of influences on physical activity: the emotional, which I had explored with disappointing results, the biological, and the social. Among the biological influences, there was the intriguing possibility that environmental temperature exerted an impact, for it had been shown to have marked effects upon the physical activity of experimental animals: lowering temperature increases physical activity, and raising it reduces activity. And obese people are unusually susceptible to the discomforts of heat and humidity. Anyone who has spent much time with obese people knows how miserable they feel during hot weather, and how even the slightest increase in body heat produced by a meal will often cause profuse sweating. For them a warm spell becomes a heat wave, when minimal physical activity produces the sweating of vigorous exercise.

Spurred by these considerations, we carried out a study which examined, among other things, the relationship of temperature to physical activity. We conducted the study at a nearby Girl Scout camp, supplying both obese and non-obese girls with pedometers: and we recorded their activity levels as heat and humidity rose and fell through the Philadelphia summer. It seemed that we could hardly fail to come up with some positive findings. In fact, I can't remember another study of which I had higher expectations.

But the results were completely negative. Neither heat, nor humidity, nor the temperature-humidity index had the slightest influence upon the physical activity of the girls. It was cold comfort to have a clear-cut negative result, but the study did help to limit our approach: we didn't need to worry about heat and humidity as causes of obesity, at least among young girls.

The next attempt to look at a biological influence on physical activity had a happier outcome, although not in the way I expected. We knew that phases of the reproductive cycle have a potent influence upon the physical activity of female rats. They will run three and even four times as far in a day during one phase of the cycle as they will in another. An influence which could be so powerful in one species must surely have some effect in another.

For a period of nearly two years I tried to show such an effect. More than 30 wives of medical students gamely strapped pedometers to their waists and recorded their activity through three or four menstrual cycles. Their activity did fluctuate wildly from day to day, but never in relation to their menstrual cycle. They did, however, show striking peaks and valleys which corresponded to another cycle—weekdays and weekends. The search for biological influences on physical activity had failed, only to lead to the identification of far more powerful ones: social factors. The largest differences in physical activity which I was to find were those between weekdays and weekends. But the differences were not always in the same direction.

Some active persons with confining jobs showed low weekday activity and a great increase in activity over the weekends, when they could give expression to their natural inclinations. Others, with little natural inclination toward physical activity, might show high levels of activity during the week, when their jobs forced them out of their sedentary ways, with a decrease on weekends. Obese people were far more likely to fall into this second category. Hyman Cohen was a shining example.

Only very rarely did Hyman Cohen walk as far on a weekend day as he did on a weekday. In fact, during the first three months of his treatment, he never did. And later, when his physical activity had stabilized at a rate of 3 miles a day, he averaged 4 miles a day on weekdays at work and no more than a mile a day on the weekends. The influence of the day of the week produced not just large differences in physical activity, but differences of an order of magnitude far beyond those produced by emotional factors. Hyman Cohen's physical activity on weekdays was four times as great as on weekends. By contrast, the increase in physical activity associated with recovery from his depression was only 50 per cent.

I meditated on these figures long and hard. The story they told was as straightforward as any I had found since I had started studying obesity. It was not a story that was congenial to the notions I had started with. For as I reluctantly began to realize, these figures made one thing clear: a simple social fact had a far stronger influence on physical activity than anything that I ever had found in the study of stress and disease.

What were other social factors that might influence physical activity? Clearly occupation was one. Our study of obese women had shown that most who gave their occupations as "housewife" were remarkably inactive. But, since most of our subjects were housewives, it was impossible to assess the influence of occupation on physical activity. It occurred to me that among men, on the other hand, the very wide spread of occupations should make it possible to do a careful quantitative study on the influence of occupation upon physical activity. So we set about the study of obesity in men.

Our very first interviews with obese men provided an interesting confirmation of Mayer's views on the importance of physical activity in the regulation of body weight. Eight of our first sample of men had served in the Army and had undergone the less than rigorous basic training of the peacetime Army. Nevertheless, they had lost an average of 20 pounds. No one lost less than ten pounds; and some lost as much as 30. Furthermore, each of these men had gained weight following basic training, and almost all had returned to their previous obese states within a few months of assignment to sedentary garrison life.

We were particularly interested in the reasons which these men gave for their weight losses and weight gains. Everyone attributed the weight loss to the increase in physical activity. None reported any conscious effort at restricting the amount he ate nor any shortage of food. All said that they had lost weight with no effort at all, eating just as much as they wished.

The accounts of these men made it clear that there was a significant increase in their caloric output during basic training. Was this increased output sufficient to account for their weight loss? Or did Mayer's discovery play a part, and did the increased physical activity result in an actual decrease in the amount they ate? And conversely, had the weight gain following basic training been due solely to a decrease in physical activity, or had there been an increase in eating?

None of the men could remember enough of the details of the food they ate to allow us to reconstruct their caloric intake. But they reported, with remarkable unanimity, that the weight loss during basic training had occurred with none of the discomfort of their other weight-loss experiences. All remembered quite well that they had lost weight despite the freedom to eat as much as they wanted. So we had clear evidence that increases in activity had not been matched by commensurate increases in eating, despite complete freedom to eat as much as desired.

It has often seemed to me that the simple observations of this group of men, obtained at so little cost, may contain more information and provide more guidance for weight reduction than other studies I have carried out at far greater expense.

After these interviews we easily and quickly carried out pedometer measurements of the physical activity of 25 obese and non-obese men. The obese men surprised us by the extent of their physical activity. On the average they walked over twice as far as the obese women—4.0 miles compared to 1.5 miles for the obese women. Furthermore, they were very nearly as active as the non-obese men, who walked no more than 4.5 miles a day. When allowance was made for the greater number of calories burned by the obese as a result of their greater body weight, it became clear that they expended just as many calories as the non-obese men.

This study thus produced another solid finding: gender

made a difference. The decreased physical activity and passive attitudes towards it, which had so clearly characterized obese women, were not found in obese men.

These differences in physical activity between obese men and women raised the question as to whether the inactivity of the women was a function of their gender or of the social influences affecting women. In other words, are obese women inactive solely because they are female or because they play a woman's role in society?

To answer this question we had carried out the study mentioned before, at the Girl Scout camp. We had measured the activity and the body weights of the girls at camp, and then again after their return to their more sedentary home life. Consequently we had the data to assess the same group in situations calling for vastly different amounts of physical activity. It looked as if we could carry out the first test in humans of Mayer's discovery with rats.

Our first question was whether the obese girls were less active than the non-obese girls; were they more like adult women or more like adult men in this respect? The results showed them to be more like the men. At home the obese girls walked 3.5 miles a day; the non-obese walked 5.0 miles a day. When allowance was made for the differing rates of caloric expenditure, the obese girls actually expended more energy at home than did the non-obese girls.

At camp all of the girls had been much more active, and the difference between the groups disappeared. The obese girls walked 7.0 miles a day, the non-obese 7.3 miles a day. The caloric expenditure of the obese girls as a result of physical activity was thus considerably higher than that of the non-obese girls.

Here was a fascinating surprise. In sharp contrast to the obese women we had studied, physical activity played no part in the obesity of these girls. How was this finding to be understood? Did it mean that the activity of obese females decreases as they pass from adolescence into womanhood? Or was our sample of obese girls a biased one, an unusual group which, unlike other obese girls, sought out the active physical and social life of the Girl Scouts? The latter alternative seemed the more plausible. But there was no way of knowing. And we turned our attention to the critical question—did a change in physical activity affect body weight? Did summer camp have the same effect as basic training?

The answer was yes! The obese girls lost weight when compared to the non-obese girls. How did this come about?

For an answer to this question we turned to ratings of appetite recorded by the girls themselves. The difference between obese and non-obese girls was striking. Most of the non-obese girls reported an increase in appetite at camp, probably in response to the increased physical activity. On the other hand, few of the obese girls reported any increase in appetite, and some even reported a decrease. Presumably the actual food intakes, which we were not able to measure, showed the same pattern.

Taken together, the findings of physical activity, appetite, and weight change provide strong support for Mayer's theory. Among the somewhat more active non-obese girls, the move to active camp life had resulted in increased appetite, presumably greater food intake, and little change in body weight. Among the more sedentary obese girls, however, the increased physical activity at camp resulted in little or no increase in appetite, presumably little change in food intake, and weight loss.

What lessons had we learned from these studies? Most important was the evid^nce that physical activity plays a part in the regulation of body weight, and not only by means of the caloric expenditure which it entails. It may play a larger part by decreasing, or at least preventing an increase in food intake, when obese people increase their physical activity.

And the level of physical activity is controlled by social factors to a far greater degree than by biological or emotional factors. Army recruits were more active and lost weight under the influence of the social pressures of basic training; the same phenomena held true for girls under the social pressure of summer camp.

Here at last were the first glimmerings of a successful

treatment for obesity. At the least they seemed more fruitful than the old preoccupation with the personal stresses of the obese. And I came increasingly to feel that social influences, more than emotional and biological, are what cause and sustain obesity.

seven
Social Class and Obesity

The work with physical activity profoundly changed my out-look. It made me aware for the first time of the vital role of social factors in the production of obesity. But another line of investigation was to change my outlook even more decisive-ly. This research focused directly on the relationship of social class and obesity. It led me still further than Harold Wolff's theories of stress and disease, with their emphasis on the life history and experience of the individual, and more deeply into the significance of broad community-wide social factors.

The inquiry began with a question which came to preoc-cupy me increasingly over the years: Are obese people more neurotic than non-obese people? By this time I was in no

doubt as to the extent of neurotic suffering among obese
people. There was a very great amount. I had treated enough
to know how disturbed they could be, and how even obese
people who seemed on first acquaintance to have few problems, could, when they felt more confident, tell hair-raising
tales of their difficulties. My question was more specific: Did
obese people have more problems than non-obese people?

The route to answering this question was a circuitous
one. It began when Harold Wolff approached me one day
in his typically serious manner: "Dr. Stunkard, I have a
question. Would it be possible for you to put together a manual
for the treatment of obesity in the Army?"

The problem had apparently started some time before
when a general had received orders to prepare to move his
division to Germany. This general had commanded troops
there during World War II, and had gained a reputation for
combat effectiveness and for the emphasis he placed on physical fitness. One evening in Washington he was discussing his
forthcoming move overseas with an old friend, who was then
a member of the Joint Chiefs of Staff. While they were reminiscing about their wartime experiences, the division commander confessed how embarrassed he felt about returning
to Germany with his current troops, so far less professional
and less fit than those he had led in combat. The two old
comrades spent some time deploring the deterioration of the
peacetime Army and its lack of physical fitness. When they
came to the subject of fat soldiers they reached unanimity—
neither could stand fat soldiers.

According to Dr. Wolff's understanding of what had
transpired, the senior general had asked why the division
commander tolerated them, and the latter had protested that
he didn't see that he had a choice. The senior general report-
edly suggested, "Why don't you *order* your fat soldiers to lose
weight? And if they don't obey the order, court martial them."

The division commander said that he would like nothing
better but that he didn't know if he could. The senior general
apparently assured him that he could, and that he would

personally do everything he could to prevent his old buddy from having to undergo the humiliation of taking fat soldiers to Germany.

Upon his return to his post the division commander apparently issued an order that all fat soldiers were to start losing weight at once. Presumably some did; and some did not. After waiting a decent interval, the division commander proceeded to court martial those who did not, on the charge of disobeying an order.

The review of the courts martial was prompt and decisive, and not favorable to the general. He was now to be subjected to the double humiliation of taking fat soldiers to Germany and having his courts martial of these same fat soldiers reversed. He called his old buddy on the Joint Chiefs of Staff, who, in turn, called the Judge Advocate General. The latter explained to the former that obesity was a medical, not a legal problem, and therefore could not be handled by means of court martial. If the senior general wanted something done about it, medical, not legal channels were the appropriate route.

This route was speedily traversed. The senior general called in the Surgeon General and asked him what he intended to do about fat soldiers. The Surgeon General, in turn, called in his staff and relayed the request. Uncertain of how to proceed, but aware that treatment for obesity was unsatisfactory, they approached the Director of Research of the Army Medical Corps for any information about new methods of treatment. Remembering that the Army was contributing a small amount of money for the study of obesity to a program under the direction of Dr. Wolff, the Director of Research called him. Finally, at the end of this long chain, Dr. Wolff spoke to me.

It was never very clear what the Army wanted. When I suggested to Dr. Wolff that I go down to talk to the research people in the Medical Corps, he quickly assured me that that wouldn't be necessary. All that they wanted was a manual on the treatment of obesity in the Army. I pointed out that it would be difficult to construct a manual without knowing more about the circumstances surrounding the obesity problem.

Dr. Wolff frowned: "Well, can't you work up something for them?" he asked impatiently. "I don't think they expect a great deal."

As I paused, uncertain as to how to respond, Dr. Wolff turned and walked away. I heard no more about the matter for a year or more.

In fact, it was not until I had accepted the position at the University of Pennsylvania and was planning to move to Philadelphia that it came up again. At that time Dr. Wolff told me that he had decided not to continue his work with the Army. He said that he thought it would be helpful for me to start in Philadelphia with sufficient research support to get a program under way; and if I were agreeable, he would recommend to the Army that this contract be transferred to the University of Pennsylvania and that I be named Principal Investigator. I had not been involved before in research funding and I welcomed the opportunity. During the spring before I moved to Philadelphia, I went to Washington to discuss the transfer of the contract with its sponsors in the Army Medical Corps.

It was a curious meeting. The two middle-aged captains with whom I spoke had not negotiated the initial contract, and they acted as if their job were simply to make sure that the technical requirements were met and the amenities observed. As to the fruits of the research, they could not have cared less. And the possibility of conducting a study with Army personnel horrified them.

"That would be quite out of the question, Dr. Stunkard."

"Why?" I asked.

The tall captain began. "Well, you don't understand our situation, what the Army's like today. It's not like it used to be. We've got to be terribly careful. We can't do anything that might offend the men. You can hardly do any kind of studies in the field any more. The first thing you know, some kid gets his nose out of joint and writes his mother, and she gets in touch with her congressman, and we have an investigation on our hands."

Anxious to protect the contract with the Army, and assuming that it was not being given as a form of charity, I tried to think of some study which would warrant continuing support. "What," I asked, "would you think of a study of obesity in men?" A good number of the obese men in any sample would be likely to have had military experience. It might well be possible to learn something about their body weight changes in relation to various aspects of military service. I quickly outlined a research project.

"That sounds like a fine idea," they replied with obvious relief; "just don't get the Army involved." They were beaming as they rose and escorted me to the door. "Thank you for coming to see us, doctor. Just remember, don't get us involved."

Thus was born the research project on "Obesity in Men." The following year, midway through the study, I received a polite letter from the Army which, in one paragraph, thanked me for past services and terminated the contract. By this time I had become so involved in the study that I carried it out anyway.

It began soon after I arrived at the University of Pennsylvania, and involved intensive work with 25 obese men, and a matched number of non-obese men who served as control subjects. We looked for distinctive personality patterns among the obese men and again returned to the question which had begun to obsess me: Are the obese more neurotic than the non-obese?

In short order we were flooded with data; and nowhere was this embarrassment of riches more embarrassing than in the analysis of the psychological testing. For until that time there had been no standard way of comparing groups on the several dimensions of psychological functioning which were assessed by these tests. As luck would have it, just at that time there appeared a book, *The Interpersonal Diagnosis of Personality*, which provided a general framework for analyzing our psychological test data.[10] Its author was Timothy Leary.

When our study was well underway, I wrote to Dr. Leary and received an invitation to visit him. We spent a pleasant morning discussing the research which each of us was carrying out. As I have since read about Timothy Leary's later life, I have often thought back to that morning and the shy, kindly man who went out of his way to be of help. He seemed pleased that we were using his system in research on obese people, and I was surprised by the deference shown me by this man, already well-established in his field and the author of one of its significant texts.

Dr. Leary described in some detail his goal of collecting a data bank containing detailed psychological tests of groups of similarly afflicted people. As I remember it, he had already collected tests on large numbers of people suffering from asthma and other psychosomatic diseases, as well as on delinquents at a reform school. He hoped that these large homogeneous groups could serve as contrast groups for researchers all over the country, who could compare their results with those in his data bank. He envisaged this bank as a kind of national resource which would make it unnecessary for each investigator to recruit his own contrast group.

I was pleased when he asked me if we would consider including our data on obese men in his bank, and I assured him that we would be glad to do so. We parted with an agreement to stay in touch and to do what we could to increase the usefulness of psychological tests.

Shortly afterwards other interests led Timothy Leary from the field of psychological testing. I also left soon thereafter, persuaded by the results of the study of obese men. After months of examining the data from every possible vantage point, the results were clear-cut and negative. The obese men showed no distinctive personality features. Many of them showed signs of emotional disturbance, but just as many non-obese men showed the same signs.

About that time I came across a remarkably similar study of obese women in a psychology journal. Its results were the same as ours. Psychological tests showed little difference between obese and non-obese women. There was good reason to give up on this line of research and to conclude that there are no psychological differences between the obese and the non-obese. But I had not completely given up hope of pursuing that quest. Perhaps, with a larger number of subjects. . . .

A new phase of the investigation began one beery evening at Atlantic City during the meetings of the American Psychosomatic Society. That afternoon one of my students had made a beautiful presentation of some of our research, and a group of us celebrated the occasion with a lobster dinner, followed by a visit to the bar of one of the large hotels which line the Boardwalk. Alive with the medical and biological research meetings that grace Atlantic City in the spring, these bars are beehives of activity, some social and some professional. We entered the hotel in search of the first and emerged with the second.

As our group moved through the dim light of the bar I spotted Leo Srole, a sociologist who had worked at the New York Hospital when I was there. He had also presented a paper that day at the Psychosomatic Society meeting, and he too was elated with its reception. We immediately got into a discussion of his research.

Leo Srole had been the director of a research group which, during the previous several years, had carried out a survey, the most carefully yet done, of the rates of mental illness in a general population. Teams of interviewers had gone into a large area around the New York Hospital and had meticulously assessed the mental and emotional symptoms of a selected sample of the population. While I had still been at the hospital, Leo had been involved in managing this massive collection of data and in preparing it for analysis. Now the first analyses were finally beginning to come off the computer, and he was harvesting the fruits of years of labor.

The most striking finding of what became known as the "Midtown Study"[11] was the very high frequency of mental and emotional symptoms in the general population. As many as 20 percent of randomly selected subjects reported impairment in family relationships and work performance, and significant symptoms of emotional distress. Srole was bubbling

over as he told about the very high levels of statistical significance of his conclusions:

"With 1660 subjects, you can just about count on definitive answers to your questions. You can hardly fail to find
something if it's really there."

The mention of the large number of subjects and getting
definitive answers jolted me. I could hardly wait to ask, "Were
your obese subjects more neurotic than your non-obese ones?"

There was a long pause.

"You know," Leo began, "We never did look at obesity."

We stared at each other.

"Well why not do it now?" I asked. "You must have
heights and weights on your subjects."

"Of course we do," Leo replied.

Since Leo did not have the time or the resources to add
this additional inquiry to his research program, he agreed
to make his data available to me. We reviewed the design
of the Midtown Study and it soon became clear that it couldn't
have been better suited for testing the relationship between
obesity and neurosis.

The first step had been to identify a population of 110,000
persons consisting of everyone between the ages of 20 and
60 living in a specific area on the East Side of Manhattan.
The area had been selected in order to include a wide variety
of social and ethnic backgrounds. It included groups from
the very lowest socio-economic status—unemployed people and
those living in poverty, old lower-class ethnic neighborhoods,
some middle-class areas, and a section of Park Avenue with
some of the most expensive housing in the city. Altogether
it included seven different ethnic groups, divided about
equally into those who were foreign-born themselves, those
with foreign-born parents, and those whose families had been
in the United States for more than one generation. It was,
in short, a microcosm of the city.

The 1660 subjects, representative of the 110,000, were
selected for the study and interviewed in their homes by
trained field workers for periods of two hours. The interviewers

gathered information about the social class and ethnic background of the subjects, about the number of physical illnesses, and about a number of psychological factors. The researchers then scored each subject on a variety of indices of neurosis: "childhood anxiety, withdrawal, neurasthenia, depression, anxiety, rigidity, suspiciousness, and immaturity."

Although they had collected the weights of the subjects and entered them on IBM cards, the researchers, preoccupied with the more pressing issues of mental illness, had not done anything with them. They were just sitting there waiting for us. And the information was perfect for answering our question. From the heights and weights of the subjects we could calculate the percent overweight of each and identify those who were obese. For each obese and non-obese person there were indices of their psychological functioning. It was a simple matter to determine whether the obese persons were more or less neurotic than the non-obese.

The answer, when it finally came after all these years, was an anticlimax. The results were straightforward enough. Obese people were clearly more neurotic than non-obese people. In seven out of eight of the psychological measures they showed higher levels of neurosis. And this was true for men and women, young and old, and for all three social classes —low, middle and upper.

The problem was that the differences were really very small. Although they were statistically significant, largely because they were based on such a large sample, they were quite insignificant from a practical point of view.

Among obese people 63 percent showed immaturity, compared to 49 percent for the non-obese; for suspiciousness the comparable figures were 43 percent and 25 percent; for rigidity, 67 percent and 45 percent; for depression, 25 percent and 18 percent.

So finally the question was answered. And, as I had half-expected, the answer brought with it no great insights nor any prescription for action. From now on we could feel secure in talking about the greater amount of neurosis among obese people. But it was not at all clear how this related to their obesity, nor what was to be done about it. In a negative sense we had perhaps contributed something: it would be difficult to find in these data much support for the theory that neurosis was the cause of obesity.

As weeks went by the study kept bothering me, much like the original question had. It wasn't clear what more could be made of the results, but I had a strong conviction that somehow something more could be done with them.

The solution came suddenly. I remember sitting at a counter in the Pennsylvania Station in New York City eating a dish of ice cream, waiting for a train back to Philadelphia. Nagging thoughts about the study kept coming into my mind. It was in a kind of reverie that I found myself thinking about the correlation between social class and mental illness, which earlier investigators had discovered and which the Midtown Study had confirmed. My thoughts continued on to a similar correlation which we had found between social class and obesity. Suddenly it occurred to me that I had never heard any mention of such a correlation any place else. And yet, if my memory was correct, the differences had been enormous.

I could hardly wait to get back to Philadelphia to look at the data. And when I did, the results were stunning. No one had ever before noted a relationship between social class and obesity, and here it was—the most powerful influence we had ever looked at, perhaps the most powerful influence we would ever find.

In the ensuing months we analyzed and re-analyzed the data, exploring the relationship between all kinds of social factors and obesity. Hardly a week went by without some fascinating new finding. Furthermore, the discoveries fell into a general pattern, which became clearer the further we went. It seemed that the nearer a group of people approached the standards of upper-class values, the less the amount of obesity.

A great deal of what we learned was summarized in a graph which showed the relationship of socio-economic status to obesity among women. When the women's own socio-economic status was considered, there was a six-fold difference

between those of lower and upper status. Obesity occurred
in 30 percent of women of lower socio-economic status, in
16 percent of those in the middle status, and in only 5 percent
of the upper status.

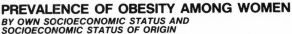

PREVALENCE OF OBESITY AMONG WOMEN
BY OWN SOCIOECONOMIC STATUS AND
SOCIOECONOMIC STATUS OF ORIGIN

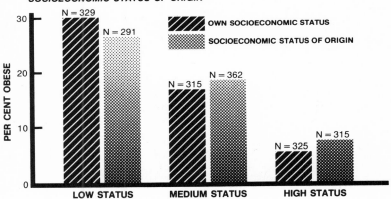

The data also allowed us to look also at the socio-
economic status of the parents of our subjects, to determine
whether social class influenced obesity, or vice versa. The
results showed that the influence went both ways, but that
social class had a far stronger influence upon obesity than
obesity did upon social class. This conclusion is seen clearly
in the graph, where the relationship of the parents' social
class to the subject's obesity is almost as strong as that of
the subject's own social class. Since the subject's obesity presumably could not have influenced the parents' social class,
their social class must have influenced the obesity.

Nonetheless, obesity did influence social class to some
degree. Another way of arranging the data shows this influence
clearly. We divided our population into those people who
remained in the social class into which they had been born,
and those who either rose or fell in social class. Of the women

who remained in the social class into which they were born, 17 percent were obese. Among women who moved downwards in social status, on the other hand, there was a higher frequency of obesity—22 percent. Among those who moved upwards in social class, the frequency of obesity fell to only 12 percent.

What does this mean? Does a subtle, or not so subtle discrimination against obese women result in their attracting only lower-status husbands and finding only lower-status jobs? Does it mean that those women who conform to upper-class standards—which prominently include thinness—are rewarded by higher-status husbands and higher-status jobs? It appears so, and others have since reported more direct evidence. One of these was Jean Mayer, who showed that attitudes towards obese people, and their own attitudes towards themselves, qualify them as still another of America's discriminated-against minorities.

Exploring the relationship of social class to obesity was only the first of our analyses. We also examined the relationship between the number of generations during which a subject's family had been in the United States and the frequency of obesity. Twenty-four percent of foreign-born women were obese, and this percentage fell steadily with the number of generations in the United States, to a figure of 5 percent for women with no foreign-born grandparents.

We then looked at the breakdown of obesity according to religion. Starting with the three major religions, we determined the frequency of obesity among Protestants, Catholics, and Jews. By this time we were not surprised by the highly significant differences, nor by the nature of the differences. Obesity was most common among Jews, followed by Catholics, with Protestants showing the least amount of obesity.

Next we turned to the breakdown between the Protestant denominations, hardly daring to hope that our luck could extend this far. But it did. The frequency of obesity faithfully mirrored the social status conventionally ascribed to these denominations. The largest amount of obesity was found among Baptists. There was less among Methodists, with Presbyterians and Episcopalians showing progressively lower rates of obesity.

The remarkable consistency of our findings up to this time led us to expect that we could also detect a pattern in the ethnic affiliations of our subjects. Long before the data began to emerge from the computer, we constructed a ranking of the different ethnic groups according to the rate of obesity which we expected. The lowest frequency, clearly, would be among subjects whose families had been in the United States for a long period of time. Thereafter we guessed that the frequency of obesity would rise steadily as we moved eastward across Europe, starting with Great Britain. Ireland, we guessed would probably show a somewhat higher rate of obesity than Great Britain, and would then be followed, in turn, by Germany, Italy, Czechoslovakia, Hungary, and a Polish-Russian group. And that was how it turned out. Only one ethnic group was out of line. Among the Czechs, for some still unaccountable reason, a surprising 34 percent were obese, the highest rate among any of the groups.

We mentioned this curious fact of the high prevalence of obesity among Czechs in a casual manner in one or two medical reports, and gave it no further thought. I was surprised, therefore, during a visit to Czechoslovakia some years later, to learn that this finding was well known among Czech medical research workers. In fact, it was being used at the time by the outstanding Institute of Nutrition in Prague as justification for further support for research in nutrition in Czechoslovakia. "If our nutritional habits are so poor that even in faraway New York, and even a generation later, Czechs are the most obese of any ethnic group," the argument went, "surely we must attack this problem in Czechoslovakia today."

By this time we had accumulated a vast amount of information on social factors in obesity. The time had come to report these matters at a medical meeting and in the medical literature. And as much as I enjoy presenting papers myself, it is nothing like the pleasure of watching a student do it. With the pride of an over-involved parent, I asked Phil

Goldblatt, who had taken the lead in these studies, to deliver our findings to the annual convention of the American Medical Association.

For days beforehand Phil worked on his presentation until it was letter-perfect, faithfully conveying our intriguing findings. He seemed quite confident about giving the paper, even after we entered the large room where five or six hundred people were seated. Both of us were reassured by the talk which preceded Phil's. It was given by a prominent professor in one of the leading medical schools, and it dealt with the psychological effects of psychedelic agents. For a time it went very well. Then as the speaker began to run out of time, he talked faster and faster, flashed lantern slides on the screen at an ever-accelerating pace, and became more and more difficult to follow. Determined to complete his paper, even after his time limit was up, the Professor continued talking, despite increasingly frantic signals from the Chairman of the meeting and obvious restlessness and murmuring from his audience. When he finally sat down, there was an audible sigh of relief.

By contrast, when his turn came, Phil spoke slowly, clearly, and to the point. He unfolded our fascinating tale in a remarkably short period of time, and then turned to its implications: "It is now apparent that obesity can no longer be viewed simply as an abnormal characteristic of the individual. It must also be viewed as one of the possible, and not too infrequent, *normal* responses of persons in certain subgroups of society to the perceived expectations of their social milieu.

"The fact that obesity is six times more frequent in lower-class than in upper-class women has profound implications for theory and for therapy. For it means that, whatever its genetic and biochemical determinants, obesity in man is susceptible to an extraordinary degree of control by social factors. It suggests that a broad-scale assault on the problem need not await further understanding of the physiological determinants of obesity. Such an assault might be carried out by a program of education and social control designed to reproduce certain critical influences to which our society has already exposed its upper-class members.

"Many of the present theories about human obesity were formulated by psychiatrists on the basis of their treatment of upper and middle-class women, for whom obesity was a severe social handicap. In other segments of society, however, obesity appears to be by no means such a handicap.

"It seems quite possible that the lack of success in the control and treatment of obesity stems from the fact that until now physicians have thought of obesity as always being abnormal. This is certainly not true for persons in the lower socio-economic population. Obesity may always be unhealthy, but it is not always abnormal."[12]

Perhaps I was biased, but the applause when Phil finished his talk seemed thunderous to me.

But for Phil there was a more immediate concern. He had had no misgivings about delivering the paper itself. But he had been worried about the question period which was to follow it. For here he would be required to respond at once to any conceivable question about his paper, including ones which might well be openly hostile. After talking over the problem, we had decided to divide up responsibility for answering the questions. We planned for Phil to join me in the front row of the audience after his talk. From there he would answer those questions which he felt comfortable about and refer the others to me.

As soon as we entered the auditorium, we realized that this strategy was going to be difficult to implement. The speakers delivered their papers from a podium at one end of a large stage. Since the only stairs onto the stage were on the opposite side from the podium, it was going to be awkward to leave the stage after the talk. Nevertheless it might just be possible, and Phil planned to try it. Neither of us knew quite what to do if he did not succeed.

The moment he finished the talk, Phil turned and started to walk across the stage to the stairs. He was met half-way across the stage by the Chairman of the meeting, who had been sitting at the head of the stairs and who now motioned him back towards the podium. As Phil stopped, the Chairman turned to the audience and announced, "I am sure that Dr. Goldblatt will be happy to answer any questions."

For an instant Phil stood transfixed, with what seemed like a look of horror on his face. But the first question came so fast that he had no time to think further about how to escape. Furthermore, it was a question which he could have answered in his sleep. "What was the overall percentage of obese persons in your study?"

Phil walked back to the podium, paused, and answered the question, and then another, and another. With each answer he seemed to throw back his shoulders and speak with more decisiveness and authority.

Then, at the end of the question period, came the climax. An older physician in the back of the room was recognized by the Chairman, and asked, "Dr. Goldblatt, I would like to know, sir . . ." He launched into a long preamble which eventually ended in some kind of question, which I have long since forgotten.

The "Dr. Goldblatt" brought Phil up sharp. Then, as the preamble to the question continued, I watched a transformation in Phil. His eyes seemed to grow wider, his eyebrows rose, his shoulders slumped. I may have been mistaken, but in my memory, his toes turned in.

Finally, the question was at end. "I don't expect that you have a definitive answer to this question, Doctor, but I would just like your recommendation based upon your clinical experience."

There was a long pause, as Phil stood staring out at the audience. Then, slowly, in a small, high voice, he said, "I don't have any clinical experience. I'm just a medical student."

This time, I am sure, the room rocked with applause.

eight
Disturbance in
the Body Image

By "disturbance in the body image" I mean the distorted picture that a person may have of the physical appearance of his own body. Such disturbances have long been known to occur in certain kinds of emotional disorders—from the chronic complaining of a paranoid individual about the size of his nose, to the delusions of severely depressed people about their bowels rotting away, and the schizophrenic patient's panicky sense that his body is disappearing. But we were slow to realize that the complaints of obese people about their bodies might be a form of disturbance in body image.

It certainly took me a long time. On the face of it, there was nothing unrealistic about the complaints of many obese people. Their bodies *were* huge, awkward and ungainly. And it wasn't until the study of "Obesity in Men"—the vain effort to save my Army contract—that an unexpected finding directed my attention to the phenomenon.

I had already observed that the intensity of obese people's dissatisfaction with their bodies varied widely, and not always in keeping with the extent of their obesity. Some of the bitterest complaints came from people, predominantly women, who were only moderately overweight, while far more obese people would seem to take a more tolerant and philosophical view of their affliction. I saw no consistent pattern, and in its absence I tended to view the self-censure as a more or less realistic response to a distressing situation.

What changed my mind was a paper on "The Prognosis in Juvenile Obesity" by Mullins.[13] Convincingly, it argued that efforts at weight reduction were less successful among adults who had been obese as children than they were among those who had developed their obesity in adult life. The idea was intriguing, and we proceeded to examine all of our subjects from this point of view. Sure enough, there was such a pattern.

Not only were the "childhood-onset obese" less successful in losing weight, they also tended to be more obese and more emotionally disturbed. Despite the fact that we examined only 25 men in this study (of which 12 were "childhood-onset obese" and 13 "adult-onset obese"), the distinction between the two groups was striking. Even in conversation, they differed. The childhood-onset obese seemed more emotionally labile, more complaining, more discouraged, more demanding. The adult-onset obese seemed more stable, more laconic, more matter-of-fact. We pursued these differences further.

Not one of the adult-onset obese men made any more than casual, realistic comments about his body. Among the childhood-onset obese men, on the other hand, 7 out of 12 complained about their bodies in extravagant and derogatory ways. Some childhood-onset obese did not complain about their bodies. But when a body image disturbance was found, it was always in a childhood-onset obese person.

Clearly disturbances in the body image of obese people represented a distinct phenomenon. Clearly it was the source of untold suffering. I decided to study it, and the one who taught me more than any other was Herbert Marx.

When he first came to see me, Herbert Marx was 21 years old, just entering his senior year of college . . . and thoroughly miserable. He was a short (5′6″), awkward young man, who walked slowly into the office, leaning backwards just a little—like a pregnant woman balancing her swollen abdomen. The folds of a double chin lay beneath what seemed a small head and youthful face, with no trace of beard on his smooth, pink cheeks. He weighed 205 pounds and was gaining rapidly.

Throughout our first meeting, in fact for a long time thereafter, Herbert seemed extraordinarily ill at ease, smiling too quickly, nodding agreement at the slightest opportunity. When he left the office at the end of our first meeting, he spoke in a manner clearly calculated to reassure me: "Well, doctor, I'm sure that we'll be finding out some very interesting things together." A perhaps modest understatement, but one which would prove prophetic.

As befitted someone who had had previous experience with psychiatric treatment, Herbert had come to our first meeting with a precise formulation of three "problems" for which he wanted help: "inconsistency, unpredictability, and going to extremes."

In talking about the first of these, he spoke in a small voice of muffled desperation. "I'm a Jekyll-Hyde character. I am somebody who can change completely within an hour. Just take, for example, a time when I might be reducing. Everything's going well. I'm trying to be with other people and doing everything that's right. Then, within a few minutes I just begin to eat, and I eat and eat and eat. And what do I eat? Only the denied foods." Seeing my puzzled expression, he explained, "Candy and pie, things like that. But that's not all. When I do this, I want to be completely alone. I feel ashamed of myself, like I have a dirty, dark secret.

"Then there's the unpredictability. I just don't have any idea when these changes are going to happen. I was living downtown this year, away from home, and for a while everything at school was going well. Then I suddenly began to eat. I fight with myself. I call myself a fat freak. I do everything I can to stop eating, but nothing works and I always end up eating.

"On top of that, I'm always going to extremes. Everything is always a hundred percent good or a hundred percent bad. There's no middle ground for me. I'm either dieting a hundred percent or gorging a hundred percent. If I break my diet, even just a little bit, then I figure that the whole day's ruined. And I feel so terrible that I curse myself mercilessly, but I go right on eating. It's gotten so this thing dominates my whole life. If I feel slighted, I don't think like other people do, 'Well, it's because I'm Jewish,' but only that I'm overweight. It's something that I can't fight back about, because I agree with people—I think that I should be despised for looking the way I do." And with a despairing sigh, he nervously motioned to his body.

As I sat listening to Herbert's barrage of self-derogation, I began to grow uneasy. I tried to slow the onslaught by asking some questions. What, for example, did he hope to get out of treatment. With that, he sat back and relaxed for the first time, and his speech, when it came, was slower and less convulsed.

"I guess I would just like to feel free and easy—not feel inferior, not always feel like I'm an outsider." But the respite was only temporary. He was soon talking about his weight again, and how he divided the whole world up into two classes, fat people and thin people. "I can't really say that I want to feel free and easy, unless I lose weight, because I worry all the time about what would happen if I weren't worrying about my weight. I mean what would happen if I didn't feel that everyone hated me? I don't know, but I guess I think I would just stop trying completely, and never stop eating and just swell up until I burst. No, it's not feeling free and easy that I want; it's getting down to 160 pounds."

It was some time before I discovered the full significance of Herbert Marx's goal of 160 pounds, since our weekly meetings were dominated by more immediate concerns. He began the third visit by arriving late, in a visibly distraught state, and launching quickly into a tormented stream of complaints. "I was good until yesterday, really I was. And then suddenly I developed the urge to over-eat—starches, candy, pie, all of the forbidden foods . . . you name it. So now my perfect record's smashed, completely shattered. And today is ruined —ruined as a perfect day, that is. So now I feel it should be a completely rotten day.

"I can't tell you how it started. I was good until after lunch yesterday. Then I went to my aunt's house, and I didn't find anyone there and got to wondering what was in the refrigerator. I kept arguing back and forth with myself and I finally ended up saying, 'You'd better get as much as you can now, before you get in control of yourself again. Here's your chance. Eat! Eat!'

"I don't know why I do all this. I'm terrified of being condemned by people for my weight. And yet of course they should condemn me. It's a despicable thing to weigh as much as I do. I'm grotesque and everyone's against me because of it. What do I have to offer anyway? A fat man. Everybody rejects me. I can tell at school they feel I'm not only fat but a greasy grind. All I can do is get good marks . . . The only hope is to get to 160."

He had tried going to the gym to play badminton during the struggle between "being good and being bad." But it had been hopeless. "I would have had to shower with all the other people, and then they would have made fun of me. And I couldn't leave to take a shower in my room, because it would have meant asking the gym teacher for permission. I hate gym teachers, and I don't ask favors of people I hate. I hate all athletes. They're jocks and I hate all jocks . . . But 160 is the magic number. If I can get there, I'll be able to shower with anyone."

He finally stopped long enough for me to ask him what weighing 160 pounds meant. He seemed genuinely surprised. "Why that was what I weighed when I had a date. I even went swimming then . . . twice."

Eventually I was able to piece together an account of Herbert Marx's weight over the years, with all its wild fluctuations, from his obese childhood and infancy, through countless successful and unsuccessful attempts at weight reduction. In all of this account the golden period had been his third year in high school, when he was 16 and weighed 160 pounds and had a date. But it had been followed by "that terrible summer," when he had started on a period of weight gain which had continued without interruption until he had reached 260 pounds.

The years before we began treatment had been characterized by increasingly rapid fluctuations in his weight. He had undergone psychotherapy the preceding year and spoke blandly of how much he had learned in the course of this treatment: "But it didn't seem to help my weight. I was 180 when I started with Dr. Wilson in the fall and 250 when I finished with him in the spring. But I don't blame him for that."

What did he blame for it? "At that time I thought, 'Well, I'm in treatment and sooner or later I'll get to the cause of my obesity. So in the meantime I'll just go ahead and eat whatever I want to and put the blame on the treatment.' Then after I stopped treatment I went on a very strict diet. It only took me seven months to get back down to 180. Then all of my good intentions just gave out." By the time Herbert Marx came to me, his eating had once again gotten out of control, his weight had risen to 205 pounds and showed no signs of stopping.

During the first months of treatment, I was able to learn something about Herbert Marx's family background. His parents had come from small Jewish communities in Eastern Europe while still children, had married young, and had soon settled into lives of bitter mutual recrimination. Much of the animosity centered around Herbert's father's occupation as a junk dealer. With increasing acidity, Mrs. Marx assailed her husband for his incompetence and his inability to "get ahead in life." She was joined in her assaults by two sisters who lived close by. Together these women dominated their extended family. Although frequently bickering among themselves, they presented a solid front toward the rest of the family—often demeaning and invariably hostile.

When Herbert's family moved to a new neighborhood and his father was unable to get a new job, the full fury of the three sisters was unleashed. And one day, when Herb was 14 years old, his father just disappeared. He never saw him again. There was just one wistful reminder: each week, without fail, there arrived at the doorstep two or three recent editions of magazines addressed to "the Marx family" in his father's handwriting, with no return address.

Not long after the disappearance of his father, Herbert's mother found a small house with an apartment upstairs and a candy store and newsstand below. And as the details of his life unfolded, I could scarcely believe the degree to which his background paralleled that of Hyman Cohen.

"Mother works extremely long hours in the store—from seven in the morning until ten at night. It's terribly hard work . . . There is a great deal of petty thievery and the customers are very hard to please. I used to help out in the store on weekends, and it was usually a mess. Mother and I were always fighting. I really don't know what we were fighting about. All I know is that there's just a lot of tension around her all the time, and I was always stealing candy and ice cream and eating it.

"I never liked the store. I always felt that it was just a petty little business, that it wasn't nice. I was always worrying about people stealing things, and I just hated the whole business. I hated it." And caught in the ugly memory, he shuddered.

About two months after the start of treatment, Herbert Marx's complaints and self-derogation began to dry up. He talked more and more often about how good he was feeling and of his hopes for the future. "I'm better, much better. I'm really doing things that I never thought I could do. Like today I left the potatoes and meat on my plate. Before, I used to feel a terrible drive to eat. Now there's hardly any drive at all.

"I even ran for the train today, and it's the first time I've done that in ages. I think it's a symbol. I used to say to myself that it would make me look like a fat fool to run.

And I'd rationalize that I probably wouldn't be able to make the train anyway. So I'd say to myself, 'Why not wait around till the next train and feel miserable?'

"But it's different now. Don't you notice anything unusual about me today? . . . I'm wearing my contact lenses. I got them last year but I never got up the initiative to use them. I figured nobody would notice. But I started wearing them over the weekend and I've worn them every day since then. What do you think?"

As the weeks went by, Herbert's weight fell, from 205 to 180, and his confidence rose. "I've passed the halfway mark on the road to 160. I know I might be wrong, but I just have this conviction that the only way people think about me is in terms of my weight. When I get below 160 I'll be very nearly perfect. And I just can't imagine anyone criticizing me or not liking me then. Of course, I might find that people will hate me because I'm Jewish, or because I'm a greasy grind and get good marks. But right now I feel that everyone will have to like me. It's inevitable."

The honeymoon phase of treatment was now in full swing. It had been gratifying, very gratifying in fact, to watch the change in this morose and hopelessly discouraged young man, to watch the growth of hope and the rise in his self-esteem. And somehow, despite his euphoria, I didn't feel as concerned as I might have over an impending depression. Perhaps it was because he soon began to use his new-found confidence to try to achieve a long deferred goal.

"Now I'm all set for the next step. Now I want to have a date. That's my next project. So I'm driving to 160. The pressure is on to get there. I know it's irrational, but that's what I weighed when I had the date in high school."

What had happened on that date, I wondered. It had seemed to mean so much to him. Why wasn't there a second one? "Basically, I guess, it was because Mother disapproved. She was waiting for me when I came back from the date and asked me what we had done, so I told her. We sat in Gladys's living room and talked. That was all. But Mother said, 'That isn't what you do on a date. You take the girl out to a movie or something.' Anyhow, she disapproved, and

I lost my ambition. And my weight went up again and I never had another date, never . . ."

But Herbert Marx was determined to change that. Right after mid-year exams, he got a job waiting on tables in a local restaurant two or three nights a week, in order to have a small fund ready for dating expenses. His mother expressed concern that this work might detract from his studies, but he reassured her with ease. And three months after starting treatment his weight had fallen to 173 pounds.

"I'm pulling out the stops. I know my goals. One hundred and sixty pounds and then a date. I say to myself, 'Let's get there. Don't let anything stand in the way.' "

He left the office looking radiant.

He did not appear for his next appointment, or the one after that. He didn't call; he didn't write. He just disappeared. So I wrote him, asking if anything had gone wrong, saying that I would like to hear from him. He didn't reply. Then, a month after his last visit, he called to make an appointment.

I was stunned to see Herbert as he walked slowly down the hall to my office, 25 pounds heavier. Bloated and bitter, he slunk into a chair and gazed at the floor. He began in a low voice, "I've been eating like a pig . . ."

Laboriously, over the next month, we pieced together the story of what had gone wrong. At first Herbert said he thought it was a matter of "simple overconfidence," as he called it. "I got to feeling so cocky about things, and I said to myself, 'Why waste your money on Dr. Stunkard? He is sincere, but you don't need him. It just kills an afternoon when you could be studying. . . .' Then I wished I had my old doctor, Dr. Wilson, someone who knew my case. I had the feeling, 'You're not qualified. You don't know enough about my case.' And then I started eating, and I didn't want you to interfere with it. When I got on a binge, nothing else mattered. 'To hell with reason . . . to hell with Dr. Stunkard . . . to hell with me. I just want to get that chocolate sundae into my belly.' "

It took another month to disentangle the issues. Overeating had started immediately after Herbert had received his mid-year grades. Although he had earned, as usual, honor grades in most of his courses, he had received a C in one. Naturally it had been disappointing, but it seemed an inadequate explanation for the remarkable reversal of his upward course. We puzzled over this question for quite a while. Then, almost gratuitously, Herbert remarked that he had called his mother the evening his grades had come out.

Her reaction had been disappointment, then outrage. How did Herbert dare to bring her this kind of grade after all that she had done for him? Was this her reward for the long hours in the candy store? This showed how right she had been about his not taking the job waiting on tables. That would have to stop.

"I just couldn't convince her that that wasn't the way things were, that the work that they based the grades on was all finished before I took the job. She just kept harping on the job, so I had to tell her I would quit it." His first binges began the next morning. Was it the grade or was it his mother's reaction which had been the agent of this change? Neither. The cause was his giving in to his mother and once again becoming her little boy.

During the next six months, plagued by incessant and recurrent eating binges, Herbert gained 50 more pounds. "It's perverse. I'm not eating just to fill my stomach, but to get in as many calories as I can. It's a furious race to see how much I can eat in how short a time. I don't over-eat the way somebody else might. It's repulsive. I'm just gorging, panting, having a bowel movement. Afterwards I feel terribly guilty and unbearably thirsty . . . an incredible thirst."

This bright and articulate young man, driven by depression, told me more about disturbances in body image than I had heard from all other sources up to that time. The linkage with depression seemed critical. During the initial three months, which had been characterized by growing euphoria, Herbert had spoken progressively less about his dissatisfaction with his body. Now, immersed in depression, he could talk of little else. By the time he returned to treatment these concerns had already acquired an almost delusional character.

"Yesterday when I was in the store trying to get some special graph paper, the sales lady said they didn't have it, even though I knew they did." He stopped and nodded with a significant look. I frowned, quizzically, and he explained, "Don't you see—she was so overwhelmed by my appearance that she couldn't think straight. She couldn't even remember what they had in stock."

The distortions didn't end there. Early in this new period of depression Herbert began to withdraw from his friends. "It just isn't fair for me to be around them. Like Jerome—he has a terrible time because he's associated with me. I've ruined his reputation; it's like being associated with a gangster."

All hopes of dating dissolved. "How can I go out with a girl, any girl? She'll hate me for being fat and mentally ill." Puzzled, I asked about the nature of this mental illness. "Obsessive-compulsive. I've been reading about it in medical books, and I know what it is."

I shook my head and smiled at Herbert and said, "You dope," in what must have been an affectionate way. He brightened for a moment and sat forward and smiled. Then he sighed and said, "But that's just your reaction, and you're paid to deal with it. You'll find that the general public isn't so tolerant of mental illness."

Nor, he was convinced, were they tolerant of bodies such as his. He kept having recurring hopes of being able to go swimming, in order to expend the calories he was now consuming so avidly. "But how can I do it? I can't let anyone see me in the nude. They would just hate me. And they would have every justification for hating me, because they would see everything I hate about myself—this (with an expression of horrified disdain) obese body of mine."

As the months went by, these hateful preoccupations with his body assumed a more and more central role in Herbert Marx's life. It was as if he felt that nothing ever happened to him except in some kind of (usually derogatory) relationship to his body. And the last remaining shreds of self-confidence were periodically shattered by experiences which reminded him of his weight. On one occasion, for example, he had screwed up the courage to ask some friends to go to the movies with him. On his way to meet them at the theater he passed a large plate-glass window of a downtown department store, and suddenly caught a glimpse of himself in it. "I was just stunned by it. I felt such loathing and hatred toward myself that I turned around and went home. I couldn't face anyone after an experience like that."

This was the first of a number of times that seeing himself in a store window precipitated such a reaction. "It's gotten so that even when I'm feeling well, just looking at myself in a store window makes me sick. It's gotten so that I'm very careful not to look by accident. It's a feeling that people have a right to hate me and to hate anyone who looks as fat as me. As soon as I see myself, I feel an uncontrollable burst of hatred. I just look at myself and say, 'I hate you! You're loathsome, disgusting, despicable.' "

These reactions to his own image in a mirror seemed so striking and so predictable that in our research on distur-bances in body image, we began to ask obese people how they felt when they looked at themselves in the mirror. The answers to this simple question were frequently as helpful as any other measure in assessing the presence and intensity of disturbances in body image. Some very obese people could look at themselves in the mirror and quite matter-of-factly describe what they saw, without any particular emotional reaction. For others, like Herbert Marx, the intensity of the disorder increased with the intensity of the depression.

I will never forget the first time that I asked Herbert to look into the mirror in my office. The mirror was so high on the wall that it was necessary for him to stand on his chair in order to see himself. After a long pause he said, "Well, there it is. And I guess I don't feel so bad about it. I feel more detached."

Encouraged, I asked if he felt that I hated him for this body which he now saw reflected. "No, I don't think so. I wonder if my feelings don't have to do with the person that's with me. You're with me and I feel all right. But if Mother was with me, I'd feel sick to my stomach. Sometimes I might have forgotten for a few minutes that I was fat, and then, all of a sudden, I'd remind myself: 'You're fat, boy, and don't you ever forget it!' It's like a brand you wear. . . ."

"And what about when you're alone?" I asked.

"It's bad then," he replied. "Almost as bad as if I was with Mother. It's funny, but I think it depends on whether I'm with someone I trust. And when I'm alone, it's like I'm with people I don't trust."

The intensity of the disturbance in body image was influenced not only by the person he was with, but also by his emotions, often with startling immediacy. This was particularly clear during the period of intense guilt which followed an eating binge. "It was really uncanny last Saturday after the binge. Beforehand people looked all right to me. They seemed friendly enough, or at least neutral. And then within ten minutes everything changed. They all began to look vicious. Everyone I saw was a threat to me. Everyone. And everyone hated me."

Some psychiatrists believe that depression consists of two separable components—helplessness and hopelessness. This distinction seemed useful in considering Herbert Marx's depression, for it seemed to involve a far greater measure of helplessness than of hopelessness. At times his description of these feelings achieved a poetic quality: "I feel that I have no direction any more, no purpose . . . I'm like a feather blowing in the wind . . . a chip of wood floating down a river. A worthless cipher . . . I have no idea what to do when I finish work at the end of the day and no idea of where to go. So I just go to my room and lie down, or else I go out and eat . . . I'm completely directionless. I can't be sure of anything any more. I don't know what I believe.

"I'm empty . . . There's nothing there. I'm just like a shadow walking around the laboratory. When I'm driving the car, it's like there's no one behind the wheel. It's not that I don't know where I'm driving to, it's just that I don't know why. I feel like going up to people and asking them what their secret is, how they know to do what they're doing. It's very lonely and very frightening."

These dark moods of helplessness were rarely paralleled by comparable feelings of hopelessness. Often the depression was punctuated by brief but fierce periods of asceticism. He would embark upon rigidly restrictive 600- and 800-Calorie diets and snarl between clenched teeth, "What I need is *real discipline.* That gym instructor was right. He should have *made* me take a shower with the others, and made me so damned embarrassed that I wouldn't eat for weeks."

And when I kept raising the possibility that he might achieve at least a measure of happiness without weighing 160 pounds, he would counter vigorously, "No, absolutely no. No possibility! I'm a criminal by being over-weight. There is absolutely no chance of being happy. I am *just not allowed* to be happy while I'm overweight. If I were happy while I was overweight, the foundations of my whole world would be shaken."

Despite the severity of Herbert Marx's depression, and despite his weight gain, I somehow felt that matters were going to improve. Perhaps I was buoyed by his reaction to our visits. "I usually wake up feeling fine on the days when I am going to come in here. And I usually feel pretty good all day and for a few hours after I see you. But then the troubles begin again."

This kind of responsiveness led me to believe that he was not as sunken into depression as he sometimes appeared to be. And I was encouraged one day at the end of a particularly lugubrious hour, when he stopped at the door, turned and said in a faint, pleading voice, "Don't let me stop treatment, Doctor, no matter how much I try."

So we continued. And the weeks went by, with Herbert complaining about his failures and inadequacies. Gradually, when these pressures abated, we were able to return to the circumstances which seemed to be perpetuating his difficulties. We examined his eating binges in as much detail as possible, paying particular attention to the circumstances which seemed to trigger them. There, in the kind of conflict which preceded a binge, we began to see the problems which pervaded Herbert's life. And, as he grew more aware, the binges themselves lost some of their frightening quality, and became vehicles for mastery.

For a long time the common elements that precipitated binges remained obscure. But eventually the insights began to come. As with Hyman Cohen, it began to appear that a period of intense discomfort preceded the binge; and also like Hyman Cohen, there were hints that Herbert's discomfort was related to feelings of having been taken advantage of and of not being true to himself.

Whatever the reason, when his weight had reached 225 pounds, it began to level off. And the intensity of his complaints began to slacken. Periods of well-being began to recur, and during them he returned to his old preoccupation with dating. Eventually he hit upon an ingenious strategy. Since he couldn't stand having a girl look at him, he decided to establish a relationship by mail. He backed and filled for a few weeks on this project, and then finally sent a latter to Gladys, the girl with whom he had had the only date of his life, almost six years before.

The following week Herbert arrived at my office exuberant. Gladys had replied with a long, friendly letter. He responded immediately, and since then had written her every day. I was pleased by this turn of events, but felt the poignancy of what was happening. "One thing that makes me feel very reassured about Gladys is that she has taken a course in abnormal psychology. That makes me more confident that she can understand me."

As might have been expected, the correspondence with Gladys marked the end of Herbert Marx's downhill course. During the next five months his depression lifted, he lost 30 pounds, and there was less and less talk about his body. When he did speak about it, it was with far less vehemence and disdain.

Early in his writing relationship with Gladys, he had worried about his "dishonesty."

"Dishonesty?" I asked.

"I'm 70 pounds heavier than she remembers me. It's dishonest not to let her know. I've just got to tell her," he explained. I said that it might or might not be dishonest not to let her know, but that if he felt he had to tell Gladys about his weight, he should go ahead, and should also tell her how he himself felt about it. When he finally did, she wrote back at once telling him she understood.

Then she began signing her letters "fondly" instead of "yours truly." He kept wondering about this. What did it mean? He began to feel that he simply had to go ahead and see her. It didn't seem quite so impossible as before. "Until you mentioned it to me, Dr. Stunkard, it just had never occurred to me that her writing might mean that she cared about me. I just thought she was interested in writing me because she had taken abnormal psychology. But you're right. Signing her letters 'fondly' must mean something." And he beamed.

As the derogatory comments about his body lessened, Herbert Marx began to do things which he had longed to do for years. Sitting down and crossing his legs he held up one foot. "See what I'm wearing? My white bucks. I've had them for over a year but never wore them for fear of looking ridiculous. And now I'm wearing them even though I weigh more than 200 pounds. That's a real victory. Just like not having to wear a sweater." And I noticed that for the first time since I had known him, Herb was in shirtsleeves. "I don't need the camouflage any more."

Even the feelings of helplessness disappeared. "I feel like I'm the boss now. I'm doing what I want to do. Almost every decision about my life is one that I make. It's an entirely different ball game."

But the matter of Gladys was still unresolved. For three months their correspondence continued, she making no moves to see him, and he still afraid to risk it. By keeping to our discussions on the topic, I was able to induce Herb to explore the remaining fears which kept him from seeing her. There were some that he couldn't even write about to her. "I don't even know what I'm supposed to do on a date. Damn it all, why can't I tell her that I'm scared to see her, that I've thought for years that women hate fat men?" And, "I always thought that if someone went out with a girl, all of his loyalty would be due to her and he couldn't do anything without her. That's how I felt, that I would have to be sort of enslaved to her and give her all my time. Like the way I feel about Mother."

Quietly, by simply not allowing our conversation to diverge very long from this issue, I kept Herb talking about a date. His confidence rose. And finally there came the day when he entered the office, sat down and grinned irrepressibly. "Well, I saw her.

"And as soon as she saw me she said, 'You certainly do exaggerate.' I knew she was talking about my weight. I was just amazed at how understanding she was. And you're right, it wasn't just because she had taken abnormal psychology."

I was particularly pleased by the nature of Herbert's sense of well-being. When I asked him about "feeling so good," he corrected me. "It isn't that I'm feeling 'so good,' it's just that I'm not feeling bad any more. It isn't like that time last fall, when I was driving towards 160 and feeling so high about it. Still, you know, I'm amazed at myself. You know the L&M advertising slogan, 'They said it couldn't be done'? Well, I keep saying that to myself, and then I add: 'But I've done it, I've gone and done it.' "

These feelings of accomplishment were mirrored in his activities. "I went swimming yesterday, and it wasn't too hard. I did feel a little scared when I went to the gym, but that was nothing compared to the feeling of success I had later. I guess I felt sort of uneasy when I thought of people looking at me. But then I just got the feeling, 'If they don't like how I look, to hell with them!' It was terrific."

Herbert's weight began to melt away. He lost nearly seven pounds in the week after he saw Gladys, and the weight loss seemed different from his other efforts. "Now I just don't have any impulse to eat. Before, I used to match my drive to reduce against the drive to eat. But it's not the same now—I don't have *either* kind of drive. There's just no desire to eat." I asked what had brought about the change, and he replied, "I feel like I'm in control of my life . . . I seem to have more respect for myself. I feel that at least one person really cares,

and believes that I'm worthwhile. You pointed that out.
Gladys must care for me if she would spend so much time
writing letters."

The first date with Gladys had taken place in the middle
of October, a year after Herbert had started treatment. He
actually saw her only three times during the following month,
but each of the dates seemed to go well, and he returned
from them happy and confirmed in his more tolerant views
of his body. "When I was with her last time I even forgot
that I was overweight. I just walked along so nonchalant and
natural that I wouldn't have known myself in the old days."

Unfortunately, this happy state of affairs was not to last
long. By the beginning of December, Herbert began to report
eating binges, and his weight, which had fallen to 200 pounds,
rose to 220 pounds within a month. At first the reasons for
these developments were unclear. Then it gradually developed
that Herbert had been having increasing difficulty in getting
a date with Gladys. If he didn't call a long time before the
date, he would find her busy; and with each rejection he
found it more and more difficult to call.

After several such incidents, I urged Herbert to ask her
if things were different. For a time he ignored this suggestion,
but finally, after one particularly close therapy hour, he ac-
ceded. "O.K. I get the point. I'll find out what's happening,
no matter how bad it is. Damn the torpedoes, full speed
ahead!" And he shook my hand as he left the office that day,
saying, "I always feel so much better when I go out of here."

The period of indecision and ambiguity was brought to
a close just before the Christmas holidays. Herbert wrote
Gladys a short, carefully composed letter asking if something
had changed in their relationship. Her answer, when it came
a few days later, had an electric, and strangely paradoxical
effect.

Herbert came to the office in the afternoon, a few hours
after having received her letter. He was smiling and said that
he felt elated. He had been turned down by Gladys because
she had become interested in another boy and wanted to go

steady with him. She said that "it wasn't because I was fat but just a question of bad timing. She said she had met this other boy just before we started to go out."

He went on in a euphoric manner: "When I received the letter I went from darkest night to brightest sunshine. I went home right away and threw away all the food I had been hoarding for a binge this evening. I think I feel this way because of the relief over knowing that it is all down in black and white now. And also because she had said that it hadn't mattered that I was fat. I really feel grateful to her, because she just rejected me as a date. But she accepted me as a friend and as a human being. So I've started a new diet, and I'm going to start calling up some of the girls I met while I was dating Gladys."

I was surprised by this reaction, and not entirely reassured by it. It seemed to have much of the elation that had characterized the first honeymoon phase of our treatment. Unhappily, these reservations proved valid. The depression, which had begun tentatively and uncertainly during the period of uncertainty over his relations with Gladys, now struck with full force; and Herbert sank into a despair as pervasive as that of the previous spring. His over-eating raged out of control, and in three months his weight rose from 200 to 267 pounds.

Herbert's first response to the loss of Gladys was to return to his old, compulsive studying during every free hour of the day and night. He seemed to suffer extravagantly; and when we discussed the way he talked about this suffering, he conceded that he might have been embellishing it. But why? The answer, when it finally came, surprised me by its directness. "Mother always said, 'God will bless you for your suffering.' "

Not long after that Herb began to reexperience an intense hatred of his body. Knowing that this problem was likely to recur, we had been on the look-out for it and for its immediate determinants. And we discovered that those were neither the over-eating, which was already in full swing, nor his weight

itself. Instead, the disturbance in body image was related to
the loss of that feeling which had become so very important
to him, the feeling of being in control of his own life.

Earlier, being in control of his life had meant regulating
his eating. Now his hopes and his goals had expanded into
more human dimensions; they included going out on dates
and being relaxed with other people. The benefits which he
had obtained from treatment now seemed almost perversely
turned against him, for his expectations of himself were now
so much greater.

Three weeks after Gladys's letter Herbert reported the
return of the disturbances in his body image. From the first,
they were intense; and, if such were possible, his guilt about
the binges was greater than ever. He found himself totally
unable to eat in front of other people, and confined his eating,
now in excessive spurts, almost entirely to his room. If he
couldn't arrange to be there, he would take his food into the
bathroom and lock himself in a stall to eat.

All kinds of casual events took on new meanings. "Today
one of my friends waved at me from across the street. He's
always been someone who has been nice to me, and so I
couldn't read hatred into his wave. But I did feel that it was
very sad." I asked Herbert what gave him that feeling, and
in a thoroughly defeated voice he replied, "He's sad because
he can feel my sadness."

As Herbert Marx's treatment moved into the second year,
the reasons for his periods of weight loss and weight gain
became clearer. The first period of weight loss seemed to have
occurred almost automatically, in response to his hopes and
illusions about treatment. The succeeding five months of
weight gain had been triggered by what seemed an almost
trivial incident, his C at mid-year, followed by his mother's
using the grade to get him to quit his job. The next cycle
of weight loss and weight gain seemed entirely dependent
upon his acceptance and then rejection by Gladys.

Over the months Herbert was able to detach himself
enough from the immediate pressures of outside events to
consider the origins of his reactions, and the special meanings

that certain experiences had for him. I was particularly interested in how his disturbance in body image had started, and how it had come to occupy such a prominent place in his life. I told him that I was baffled as to how anyone could so consistently disparage himself and his body, and could not understand how this disorder had come about. Eventually we found out.

Herbert was discussing a visit home shortly after Gladys's letter of rejection. He told how his mother had spent a great deal of time telling him about the visit of the child of a relative. "All she talked about was how little the child ate. She just went on and on about how it wouldn't eat. Finally I called her on this. I asked her what she was getting at. And then she told me. She said, 'I am sorry to have to say this to you, Herbert, but I hate all fat people and I always will.'

"I was stunned by this and she probably noticed, but she went right on. She said that everybody in the family hated fat people, they just *hated* them. She got all wound up about it and told me that the only reason she had ended up with a schlemiel like my father was because she was fat and nice men didn't want her. She said that she had weighed 160 pounds then, and that was bad enough, but it was nothing to what I looked like now.

"I got terribly upset, and then she told me that she prays night and day for me to be happy. That just made me feel more guilty. The only thing she wants in life is for me to be happy, and I'm not happy, so I'm letting her down."

I asked Herbert why he thought that he wasn't happy. "How can a person be happy when he's fat? I know that just as well as Mother does."

I didn't leave the matter there. How could his mother, I asked, be so solicitous of his happiness as to pray night and day for it, while at the same time hating all fat people? Wasn't this inconsistent? Herbert left the office that day, puzzling over this question.

To my surprise and pleasure, he went straight home with it. He reminded his mother about her statement that she hated all fat people and then asked her how this applied to him.

Her response was prompt: "You, I love—all the rest, I hate."
Then he raised the question of his unhappiness. Why did
she think he was unhappy?

Apparently his mother answered, as if it were the most
natural thing in the world, "Because it's impossible to be
happy when you're fat." When Herbert told me this, I reminded him of similar sentiments coming from his lips not
too long before. He frowned, and then nodded in agreement.
Together we began to gather evidence to reconstruct the
origins of his hatred for his body.

At times he would even solicit this evidence. "Over the
weekend I decided to face her again. I went in and asked
her to tell me again how she felt about fat people. She said
that she couldn't help it, but that she just *hated* fat people.
Then she got carried away. She said that fat people were
pigs, and they ought to wear signs on their front and back
saying 'I am a pig!' "

One Saturday evening Herbert and his mother had gone
out to dinner, and things had gone well for a while. But as
soon as the waiter had set down the butter, his mother reached
over and grabbed it away. He felt disappointed, angry, and
hurt, then soon afterwards, restless. ". . . And when we were
walking home, Mother wanted to hold hands with me. This
made me feel even worse. I don't want her to treat me like
a date.

"I got away from her as soon as I could, and then I
just found myself eating . . . all sorts of forbidden foods—candy,
soda, ice cream, hot dogs. I hated every bite. It was nauseating,
just an automatic gobbling down of the food and wanting
to get out of there. I felt that I just *had* to do it. And I didn't
enjoy it at all. It was like a nightmare. I felt furious at Mother.
I kept thinking that she shouldn't have done it. I kept thinking
about how she said fat people ought to wear signs on their
front and back that say, 'I am a pig.' I just couldn't shake
it loose. And it felt like everyone on the street was looking
at me and was my enemy. So I slunk off home and went
to bed. I hardly slept at all."

During this period when we were paying special attention
to his mother, Herbert commented about her unhappiness

and discouragement, epitomized by her old refrain: "I've no Mazel [luck] . . . The world's against me." These words, I remembered, were the same ones Herbert himself had used. I also remembered that, at the time he had used them, he hadn't seemed as hopeless as the phrases implied. Here, perhaps, was the reason—they were a kind of verbal behavior taken over from his mother and used to express unhappiness, but not the deeper despair which they suggested.

As we began to accumulate more and more evidence bearing upon the sources of his difficulties, Herbert threw himself into the search with increasing enthusiasm. It didn't seem to reduce the intensity of his depression, but we did learn more and more about the historical origins of his vulnerability. And in the course of our probings he became less vulnerable. I remember with pride the day that he came into the office with a firm, angry step and threw on my desk a letter he had received the previous day from his mother. It was a short note, telling him that he was a terrible disappointment to the people who loved him, and asking why didn't he appreciate their love?

Hers was a pathetic scrawl, and under other circumstances I might have pitied the agony behind it. But I was too busy glorying in Herb's response. "What the hell does she think she's doing, sending me letters like this? It's the same old game, and I'm through playing it. She can just go to hell with her love. That's what she can do with it."

It was hard to say why, but it seemed that just at this time, when Herbert was beginning to gain some understanding of how his upbringing had warped him, his mother and aunts escalated their complaints. It may simply have been their response to his continuing weight gain. But I began to wonder if, in some subtle manner, he was not beginning to convey to them his growing disinclination to play the part they had always assigned him. In any event, the assaults continued; and we studied them and learned how he had been hurt. And he began to talk about fighting back.

Liberation was not easy. If Herbert didn't respond to his mother's pleas, an aunt could be counted on to keep up the pressure. "Yesterday one of them said to me, 'If you could only see yourself as others do. You just don't know what you are doing to yourself.' " Herb pounded his hand on the table and said that he damned well did know what he was doing to himself, and why couldn't they let him alone? "If you can't like your own body, what can you like? I've always felt different and *bad.* They keep telling me I'm no good and I agree with them. They're always saying, 'You're just like your father.' And nothing could be worse than that. He's the devil in that family."

He was able to trace back to his family the genesis of some of the fears which were keeping him from dating after his break-up with Gladys. "I keep being afraid of what a girl would think about this feminized anatomy of mine—my big hips and chest. My aunt is always talking about it. She says, 'Your breasts are larger than a woman's,' and 'your stomach is fatter than a pregnant woman's.' You can imagine how that makes me feel. It makes me feel lower than a snake. But if I were to get infuriated and walk away, they would call me a coward and yell after me, 'The truth hurts' . . . and things like, 'See? He's running away . . . just like his father.' It makes me feel like I'm evil, the most terrible person that ever lived. I don't hang around and let them do that to me any more, but still that's the way I think about myself when I'm feeling badly."

As Herbert continued to recount the seemingly endless disparagements to which he had been subjected, I began to wonder how he had been able to control his resentment over the years. Why was it that he seldom showed any resentment of their constant battering? He explained it quite simply: "Until recently I always thought that they were right and I was wrong. And I guess I still do feel that way when I'm around them. It's just in here that I begin to think that maybe I'm not wrong all the time, and maybe they don't have the right to talk to me that way.

"They're always telling me, 'You're killing your mother,' and I know how upset I can make her. I don't know whether I really think I'm killing her or not; but it's all so frightening that I guess I feel I should think whatever they tell me to think. I don't know. . . ."

Not long afterwards, when he was telling me about further disparagements by his aunts, I asked him how this made him feel. Suddenly the old tired mood was gone. He looked angry, and he said, with an outraged intensity that I had never before heard from him, "I'll never allow them to do this to me again."

Less than two weeks later, Herbert put this promise into action. It was early in the spring, at a family meeting at the house of an aunt and uncle, where he was planning to spend the summer. As far as he was concerned, the living arrangements had already been confirmed. During the course of the evening, his uncle, who was somewhat of an outsider and knew it, attempted to curry favor with his two sisters-in-law. Announcing in a loud voice that Herbert's weight was just too much for him to take, he went on to say that Herbert couldn't live in their house unless he had lost 50 pounds by June (only two months away).

"I felt very cold and very angry," Herbert reported in icy tones. "I just said, 'Very well then, I'll find some place else to live.' And I left the house, and for once in my life I didn't feel bad."

Within a month Herb had screwed up his courage sufficiently to take on his aunts. The encounters were usually brief and ugly, and were followed by long silences, or by an attempt by one aunt to intervene on behalf of the other who had been engaged in the latest conflict.

As Herbert approached independence from his mother and aunts, I expected a period of dieting and weight loss. But he lost little weight. The effects on his body image were, therefore, thrown into bold relief. He still weighed 260 pounds on the summer afternoon when, after telling me how he was increasing his social life, he said, "You know, I don't seem at all worried about my body any more. As I walk along now, I feel as though I am very light on my feet. It's absurd, I know, but it's almost as though I weigh 140 pounds." As the summer wore on, this feeling deepened. He began to wear Bermuda shorts and colorful sport clothes. Greatest of all triumphs, he went swimming. He had, in fact, reduced, but he still weighed 240 pounds when he said, "It's gotten so that

I almost *feel* thin. It's a completely different way I feel about myself, and it doesn't have anything to do with how much I weigh. I feel that I'm in command now."

Gradually, over a period of years, he began to lose weight, and the remarkable freedom from concern with his body continued. Occasionally, following a particularly painful event (which was usually coupled with an eating binge), some of the old feelings would return. But in spite of weighing over 220 pounds for the next year and a half, his disparagement of his body seemed gone. "I just can't get over it. I feel so good. It's as if my mind says that I'm not overweight, but when I look at my body it says I still am. I said 'still' because it seems to me like a cultural lag that I'm still fat. I really ought to be thin now, and I will be in a while, and it surprises me to realize that I'm not."

After all the ups and downs of this treatment, with Herbert still weighing 20 pounds more than when he first had come to see me two and a half years before, I should have been skeptical of his optimism. Curiously enough, I wasn't. I had come to believe in this young man. And although I still didn't know how he was going to do it, I shared Herbert's confidence that he would lose the weight. What became of our prophecy is saved for the next chapter.

In the meantime, I would like to tell something of the systematic studies which complemented this more intensive study of one man. I thought I understood how Herbert's disorder had developed, something about the circumstances which alternately exacerbated and alleviated it, and, finally, how it might be successfully treated. But how common were such disturbances and how often were they so severe? Which of the circumstances that seemed to have caused Herbert's disorder were peculiar only to his difficulties and which were more general? Was the disorder ever relieved by weight reduction? And what about the provocative suggestion from the earlier study of 25 obese men that these disturbances were found only among people who had been obese since childhood?

With these questions in mind, my colleagues and I studied in some detail 74 obese people. Our conclusions were summarized in a paper which was published in the *American Journal of Psychiatry.*[14]

As we had suspected, body image disturbances did not occur in emotionally healthy obese people. In fact, we found them in only a minority of neurotic obese people. Seventeen of the 74 patients in our study showed severe body image disturbances—and all of these were people who had become obese during childhood or adolescence. It was clear that their disturbances in body image were different from those which occur in brain-damaged and schizophrenic people, or in normal people under the influence of drugs, hypnosis, and fatigue. They resembled instead the disturbances reported by people suffering from deformities of parts of their body, such as deformities of the face, breasts and genitals.

The main feature of the obese person's disturbance was the constant preoccupation with obesity, often to the exclusion of any other personal characteristic. It made no difference whether the person was talented, wealthy, or intelligent; his weight was his overriding concern, and he saw the entire world in terms of body weight. Such patients often divided society into people of differing weights, and then responded to them in terms of this division: envy toward anyone thinner and contempt for those who were fatter. At the center of this attitude was the appraisal of his own body as grotesque, even loathsome, and the feeling that others viewed it with only horror and contempt.

When body image disturbances did occur, their intensity fluctuated widely, even over short periods of time. When things were going well and a person with a body image disturbance was in good spirits, he was troubled little or not at all by his disability, although it was rarely far from awareness. Let things go badly, however, let a depressive mood ensue, and at once all of the derogatory and unpleasant things in his life would become focused on his obesity, and his body would become the explanation and symbol of his unhappiness.

Despite these short-term fluctuations in intensity, body image disturbances persisted with remarkably little change over long periods of time and in the face of wide variation in life's circumstances. Weight reduction, for example, ap-

peared to have little effect upon the disturbance, a finding
which surprised and dismayed a number of obese people.
Neither the extent of the weight reduction nor its duration
seemed able to correct the disturbance in body image. And
I have yet to hear reports of spontaneous remission of the
disorder.

We also discovered that the intense self-consciousness
which Herbert Marx exhibited was commonplace among the
patients with body image disturbances. Almost all of them,
like Herbert, had serious difficulties in relationships with the
opposite sex. One attractive young woman, who in other days
would have been considered pleasingly plump, put her despair
in dramatically succinct terms: "Who'd want to marry an
elephant?" Another woman said that her body made her feel
embarrassed with men whom she thought were "normal." "So
I tend to pick up abnormal men. I tend to hang out with
fairies. That way I don't feel I have to compete with real
women."

As sad as these stories were, the study itself was satisfying.
For it refined our oversimplified views of the problems of obese
people. The more I learned about the subject, the more I
came to realize the importance of being as specific as possible
in relating neurosis and obesity. Many obese people have
severe neurotic problems. It has all too often been inferred
from this fact that the neurosis is a cause of the obesity—and
this inference is quite unjustified.

The examination of adult-onset obese people revealed
some who were severely neurotic, but whose neurosis did not
explain (nor was it even relevant to) their obesity. They could
undergo severe mid-life depressions, in response to business
reverses or family turmoil, without in any way becoming
concerned about their obesity, or even showing any change
in their eating patterns or body weight. Any understanding
of the relationship of neurosis to obesity requires careful description of which neurotic features are specific to obesity and
which are not. The disturbance in body image is one such
specific feature.

During the years since these first studies of body image,
I have tried to investigate this problem whenever the opportu-

nity has arisen. One such opportunity was provided by a fascinating study which has been under way in Hagerstown, Maryland, since 1937. It has produced startling and disturbing data on the body weight of the 100 children who had been identified as obese in 1937 (when they were 12 years old). Only 17 of these were of normal weight as adults!

Some time after first learning of this study, it occurred to me to try to study some of the members of this unique group. I went to Hagerstown and was able to locate 10 of the 17 people who had been obese as children but of normal weight for over 20 years. How did they feel about their bodies?

Three of the ten, all women, reported the onset of body image disturbances during adolescence and their persistence to the present time! Twenty years after weight reduction, all three women reported undue and morbid preoccupation with their physical appearance, and anxiety, often intense, over the gain of even two or three pounds. All of them said that they had to diet constantly.

These three people showed similarities which clearly distinguished them from the seven people who were not afflicted with disturbances of body image. First, all three were women. Of the remaining seven, only one was a woman. These three, and only these three, reported that their weight reduction had been undertaken for cosmetic reasons and in large part as a response to external pressures, such as teasing about their obesity. All reported that their weight reduction had occurred during late adolescence and had been the result of a conscious and deliberate effort. Only one other subject, a man who had reduced at age 28 for medical reasons, had lost weight deliberately.

The contrast between the three women and the six men was striking. None of the men had been particularly concerned about his obesity, nor had he made any effort to control it. Four said that they had just "outgrown" their obesity during adolescence, usually in connection with a job which required heavier work than they had been accustomed to. For two others the association with obesity was so casual that they said they did not remember having been overweight as children.

This small but select group taught us a good deal about the determinants of body image disturbances in obesity. First, the experience of these people made it seem that adolescence was the critical time for the genesis of these disturbances. None of the three women had been obese after the age of 19, but by this time each had developed a clear-cut disturbance in body image. Second, these disturbances were confined to people who had been subjected to external pressures (most commonly teasing about their weight), and who were vulnerable enough to these pressures to attempt weight reduction. Third, even this short experience during adolescence had left scars which were clearly present over 20 years later. Fourth, all but one of the subjects who remembered when they had reduced had done so during adolescence. Finally, only 17 percent of the obese children were normal-weight adults; 83 percent were not. The odds against an obese child's being a normal-weight adult were more than four to one. And for those who did not reduce during adolescence, the odds may have been more than 28 to 1.[15]

These studies provide strong evidence that the disturbances in body image of obese people have their origins during a relatively short period of time—when emotionally disturbed adolescents incorporate the derogatory views of peers and parents into enduring views of the self. Earlier observations had prepared us for these findings. Ethologists have described so-called "critical periods" during which specific influences have a decisive effect in "imprinting" various kinds of behavior. This kind of consideration was implicit in the psychoanalytic theory of personality development, and Freud's recognition of the crucial role of early childhood experience may well have been the first systematic exposition of the concept of "critical periods."

We do not have to look far for the frustrations of obese adolescents. Almost all report heart-breaking accounts of the pervasive ridicule to which they have been subjected. Indeed the pattern of discrimination against obese adolescents is so intense and far-reaching, that they could well qualify as a (heretofore unrecognized) minority group.

A brilliant series of recently conducted studies of fat tissue have helped to explain the remarkable persistence of child-hood-onset obesity and the special characteristics of people suffering from this condition. These studies, by Jules Hirsch at the Rockefeller University,[16] have shown that animals and people with childhood-onset obesity have a greater number of cells in their fat tissue than do those with adult-onset obesity. Over-feeding in early life results in both an increase in cell size *and* in total number of fat cells. When an animal is made obese in adult life, on the other hand, he grows no new fat cells; the ones he has simply enlarge.

An adult with juvenile-onset obesity may have five times as many fat cells as one whose obesity began in adult life. With weight reduction, individual cells shrink greatly, but the total number of cells remains constant. The special character of the fat tissue of childhood-onset obese people sets them apart biologically from their adult-onset counterparts. And the special character of this fat tissue may well mean that reducing to so-called "ideal weight" by adult-onset and child-hood-onset obese people have quite different consequences. The fat cells of the adult onset obese may simply be reduced to a normal size, while the far more numerous fat cells of the childhood-onset obese are being severely depleted of their fat stores.

The more I have thought about the implications of Hirsch's work, and reviewed my experience with childhood-onset obese people, the more I have wondered whether at least some degree of overweight on the part of these people may not be normal for them. They can achieve weight loss to statistically "normal" levels—but perhaps only at the cost of living in a state of semi-starvation. Small wonder that they have emotional problems and are vulnerable to depression.

We will leave the problem of disturbances in the body image at this point. It has been a satisfying problem to study. First, there was the satisfaction of coming to grips with it in the course of treating a particular patient. Then, a more systematic study helped to define the problem further. Finally, for the first time in my work on obesity, there has been a convergence of psychological and biological research, as studies of fat tissue help us to understand the disturbances in the body image. The Herbert Marxes of the future may not be as alone in their pain.

nine
Psychotherapy and Obesity

The ultimate concern of physicians—whatever they may do and however far they may stray from it—is treatment. This concern, perhaps more than any other, distinguishes physicians from scientists. Admittedly their interests may converge, and they are frequently dealing with the same issues. But the two approach their work with clearly distinctive goals.

The scientist is ultimately interested in knowledge, and theoretically there is no limit to the extent of his inquiry. In fact the quest of the scientist never stops. Each new discovery gives birth to a new theory, which suggests a new discovery . . . and so on, without end. The eventual aim of the physician, on the other hand, is to make a decision; and the better the physician, the more he seeks to know. But, in distinction to the scientist, there is a point at which his search must stop. Using the information available, he must act on it.

The most important decisions that a physician makes are those about treatment. Thousands of times each day in the United States, physicians reach critical judgments about treatments for obesity. And every year tens of millions of Americans attempt weight reduction.

Of course the doctor's office is no longer the sole province of dieting advice. With enormous fanfare, new schemes for weight reduction are constantly turning up in magazine articles and how-to books. The paths to slenderness seem countless. There are high-protein diets and low-protein diets, high-carbohydrate diets and low-carbohydrate diets, high-fat diets and low-fat diets, rice diets and banana diets, the "drinking man's" diet, and the "prudent" diet, and even (defying the laws of thermodynamics), a diet in which we are told "calories don't count." Fasting has come into considerable vogue, as have appetite suppressants like the amphetamines, and exercise programs of one strenuous sort or another.

Some of these regimens are harmful; others are not. Any given approach may be successful for one person (at least in the short run), but useless or even disastrous for another. Basic to most, however, is the unrealistic notion that there is a cure-all for obesity. We are led to believe that weight loss is a simple matter: it requires only the reduction of caloric input to levels lower than output. And, in the last analysis, that is true. But its very simplicity leads to an illusory sense of ease about the task. It should be easy. But is it? What are the results of medical treatment for obesity?

Repeatedly, we have learned the distressing answer: Most obese patients will not enter medical treatment for obesity; of those who do, most will not lose a significant amount of weight; and of those who do lose weight, most will regain it.

What about psychotherapy? Has it proven any more successful than these other methods? Again, the findings are disheartening. *Obesity is a chronic condition, resistant to treatment and prone to relapse.*

Of course information about reducing diets is so widely available that only people who have already failed to lose weight on their own come to the doctor's office. And only the failures from medical treatment reach the office of the psychiatrist. In this context it is perhaps easy to understand why psychotherapy seems to have been no more effective than other, less expensive, aids to weight reduction. Less understandable is the widespread belief in the effectiveness of psychotherapy. Many people are convinced that it is the only truly definitive treatment for obesity. There is no evidence to support this belief.

It is my belief that psychotherapy *cannot* change the basic pattern of over-eating in response to the stress that is so common among obese people. Years after even successful psychotherapy and successful weight reduction, people who have over-eaten under stress continue to do so.

Does this mean that psychotherapy has no place in the treatment of obesity? Decidedly not. Although in all probability the pattern of over-eating in response to stress cannot be changed, psychotherapy can help obese people live less stressful and more gratifying lives. When this occurs, they are less apt to over-eat. They may even reduce and stay reduced.

These benefits are no less significant for being nonspecific results of treatment. Furthermore, psychotherapy may be quite effective in controlling two specific conditions: disturbances in the body image and binge-eating. Both have been successfully treated, and patients suffering from them have achieved enduring weight losses. Neither has been influenced by other forms of treatment (including, as we have seen, weight reduction). But psychotherapy of patients with these conditions may require years to ensure lasting results.

The first question to be answered concerning psychotherapy, and one which is all too often left unresolved, is whether it should be undertaken at all. My earlier experience with dieting depressions had driven home the fact that psychotherapy is not necessarily harmless. As is perhaps true of any kind of treatment, the capacity to heal may carry with

it the possibility of harm; and the decision to undertake psychotherapy requires careful assessment of the likelihood of
each outcome. For even when there is no outright harm,
treatment can bog down in a prolonged and painful therapeutic impasse. The patient may receive little or no benefit,
and his energies and attention may be diverted from more
rewarding activities in the real world. For patients and therapists caught in such impasses, it is often difficult even to
recognize the problem, let alone terminate treatment.

The psychotherapist's first step in determining whether
treatment should be undertaken is to find out from the patient
what he considers his problems to be, his strengths in coping
with these problems, and what he hopes to gain from the
treatment. In the course of learning about these matters, the
psychotherapist also usually learns a great deal more about
other matters, of which the patient himself is not fully aware.
The critical judgment as to whether to undertake treatment
should depend in large measure upon the therapist's assessment of his ability to help the patient achieve reasonable goals,
without undue risk and without excessive investment of time
and effort.

The importance of an early agreement between patient
and therapist upon the goals of therapy cannot be overstated.
I expect that psychotherapy has come to grief over a failure
to reach such agreement during this initial period, as frequently as from any other problem. Conversely, psychotherapy
has often been carried out successfully in the face of forbidding
odds, largely because of a clear contract between the patient
and the therapist as to what they were proposing to do.

My initial conversation with Herbert Marx left me uncertain as to the degree to which we had achieved, or could
achieve, agreement on goals and expectations. Many of the
signs were favorable: Herbert's earlier psychotherapy had
helped him to think systematically about his problems, and
his initial formulation of them was reasoned and thoughtful.
All three complaints which he formulated—"inconsistency,
unpredictability, and going to extremes"—were clear and disturbing kinds of behavior; and he described them and the

associated difficulties articulately and well. Within a short period of time I was able to construct in my own mind a sense of how he viewed himself and his world.

I could even feel his sense of being an indulged and helpless child who had really only one task in the world—to control his eating and his body weight. Success in this task meant continuation of a warm and happy life. And the task seemed, on the face of it, to be a simple one. But to Herbert's distress, mysterious forces always seemed to sweep in upon him, to overwhelm him and force him to over-eat and gain weight despite his every effort. The result was estrangement from everything he held dear, and his descent into a world of misery and self-hatred.

Because of this pervasive self-derogation I approached the effort to define our treatment goals with some uneasiness. But his first definition was reassuring: "I guess I would just like to feel free and easy—not to feel inferior, not to always feel like I'm an outsider." I was moved by this honest, human wish. It seemed like a realistic goal, and one which I expected he would work hard to achieve. I felt the same way about his more specific goal: dating Gladys. Beyond that, I liked Herbert from the first. And, as recent research has shown, the therapist's liking for his patient is as important to the outcome of treatment as are his positive expectations. Both are predictive of success.

Another important predictive factor is the degree to which the patient can relate his symptoms and his disturbed behavior to specific problems in his life. Since a great deal of psychotherapy involves discovering just such relationships, evidence that the patient has some native ability bodes well for the outcome of treatment. If, on the other hand, the patient comes to treatment with no apparent ability to see connections between his problems and his symptoms, he isn't likely to develop it during treatment. To some degree every neurotic person has failed to make such connections, and Herbert Marx was no exception. His description of the way in which the impulse to eat would arise out of the blue and suddenly overwhelm him conveyed his mystification as to what was

happening to him. I had the sense, however, that down deep
he had at least a rudimentary understanding of his difficulties.
He showed no hesitancy in relating his "loss of ambition to
date" to his mother's unfavorable response to his date with
Gladys. And he spoke with some insight into the origins of
"the terrible summer" when his weight had risen from 160
to 260 pounds.

But, beyond these proofs of awareness, there was another
element that influenced my assessment. In trying to predict
the prospects for a patient entering psychotherapy, I have
generally placed a good deal of importance on certain kinds
of incidents, incidents which show that the patient's symptoms
or disturbed behavior can be interrupted by some kind of
human contact. At the time of his second visit, Herbert reported one such episode which moved me deeply and gave
me greater hope for his treatment than I otherwise might
have had. Each of us referred to it at times, and it became
a source of comfort to us both during dark periods.

About the time Herbert had started treatment, he was
accepted into the graduate program of a local institute of
technology. But this good fortune had had no effect upon
his misery or his over-eating, and he had dismissed it with
a shrug when I complimented him about it. Then, the day
after his second visit to me, he over-ate during the morning,
and ". . . I decided to really go out and ruin the day. I was
just leaving Mother's house to go down to the bakery to get
some food and start bolting it down when I met Ruth. She's
a neighbor of my mother's, and she's a freshman at Drexel.
When she saw me, she came right up and congratulated me
on getting accepted into the graduate course, and then she
welcomed me into the Drexel community.

"What happened next was really amazing. By the time
I got in the car I'd decided against starting on a binge, and
so I drove on down the street and past the bakery. I had
the thought, 'It's not too late. You still have friends!' My
optimism started to return. So I drive on to the drugstore
and bought a roll of film instead."

I asked Herbert if anything like this had ever happened before, and he said he thought so, but rarely. "I hardly ever see girls at all any more. I feel even more inferior around girls than I do around boys. But then I felt, 'Well, at least one girl accepts me.' And it didn't take more than a minute to call off the binge."

I remember marveling at the time about how one of Herbert's voracious eating binges could be aborted by such a small human event. It gave me hope. I felt that if such a small show of human kindness could interrupt his agony so decisively, somehow I would have to help him to become better acquainted with this sort of experience.

Once having decided that the prospects of success in psychotherapy are sufficiently high, and the probability of injury to the patient sufficient low, what do we do when we we undertake psychotherapy? What is it that happens in the process?

Ever since I read Jerome Frank's insightful volume, *Persuasion and Healing,*[17] I have been influenced by its thesis that psychotherapy consists of two distinct and clearly separable elements. One, "persuasion," consists of learning new forms of behavior and new outlooks on life which are more adaptive to the situation in which the individual finds himself, and more useful in coping with its stresses. "Healing," on the other hand, consists primarily of an increase in feelings of well-being and self-esteem, along with decreases in unpleasant emotions, particularly anxiety and depression.* Whereas persuasion usually requires a certain minimum exposure to the therapeutic process, healing may occur within one visit; and, in fact, it is unlikely to occur at all if it does not begin promptly.

---

*The phenomenon of healing is particularly well exemplified in the so-called "placebo" response. A placebo (from the Latin, "I will please") is a biologically inactive substance, which, when administered to a patient, relieves his symptoms. The effectiveness of placebos in the relief of all manner of symptoms, some physical as well as psychological, has been known for centuries. Indeed, until the advent of biologically effective medicines during the past half century, the history of medicine was very largely one of the placebo effect.

Whereas persuasion exerts its effect largely through its influence upon our reason, healing contains a sizable component of irrational elements. Both processes depend to some degree on the skill of the therapist, but healing seems a far more capricious event, and more contingent upon the personal qualities of the therapist.

What goes on in psychotherapy? There must be as many conceptual schemes elucidating psychotherapy as there are therapists, and it is difficult to find a basis for choosing among them. One which appeals to me sees psychotherapy as a composite of five processes or operations: (1) the use of a special kind of personal relationship to (2) discern the problems, and the strengths, of the patient, to (3) isolate the various elements of the problems, and to (4) devise strategies for coping with these elements and helping the patient implement these strategies, with success leading to (5) increased mastery, especially in personal relationships, with an associated elevation in self-esteem and decrease in painful emotions. This scheme helps to describe what occurred during the treatment of Herbert Marx.

As discussed in the previous chapter, the first three months of treatment were spent in a "honeymoon" phase. This period of heightened mood and lessened anxiety is common in all forms of psychotherapy, and is very gratifying to both patient and therapist. Of the two elements of psychotherapy, persuasion and healing, the honeymoon consists largely of healing. Like healing in general, it is poorly understood. In any event, obese people seem no more likely to experience a honeymoon phase of treatment than do the non-obese. Factors other than obesity determine the intensity of the honeymoon and, in fact, whether it occurs at all. Loneliness, for example, must be a powerful stimulus. Desperation, feelings of helplessness, and a sense of personal ineffectiveness all have comparable effects.

Given the predisposition of a patient to experience a honeymoon, what other elements are needed? A critical ingredient, perhaps *the* critical ingredient, is the evocation of hope.

It seems to be always present in honeymoons, and absent when a honeymoon does not occur. Patients frequently comment that the early evocation of hope springs from a sense that order is being brought out of the chaos of their lives. Previously inexplicable and depressing reactions of their own and of other people become understandable. They find themselves able to cope with problems which had formerly overwhelmed them.

Such was the honeymoon phase of Herbert Marx's treatment. His first formulation of his problem, in terms of inconsistency, unpredictability, and going to extremes, started the process. There seemed no doubt that the unpredictability of his responses, particularly his eating binges, was a major factor in his profound sense of helplessness. By defining unpredictability as a problem, he narrowed the distressingly large and variable field of painful events to one general class. And he thereby helped to define the nature of our therapeutic task.

One of the major contributions to bringing order out of chaos was to review with Herbert the circumstances of his family life. Prior to these discussions he had been strongly inclined to attribute his unhappiness solely to his inability to control his eating. He seemed quite unaware that the kind of assault which had driven his father out of the family might also have led to his feelings of inadequacy and self-hatred. The notion that his difficulties were not entirely self-inflicted, and that the actions of other people contributed to them, was a source of enormous relief. The discovery that other people could also affect his feelings of well-being, and even play a role in the control of the mysterious and terrifying eating binges, was just as important. For he had exhausted his attempts to regulate his life by controlling his eating, and it was reassuring to learn that his problems lay in his relationships with other people—that they could be dealt with by changing those relationships.

The occurrence of at least a small honeymoon in the form of decreased anxiety and heightened self-esteem is, I think, indicative of future success in treatment. Its occurrence

does not insure such success, as was so dramatically demonstrated by the dieting depression. But when a honeymoon
fails to develop, treatment is far less likely to be successful.

The honeymoon seems to derive much of its potency
from the special personal relationship between therapist and
patient. Of course the end of the honeymoon doesn't in any
sense mean the end of this special relationship. It may, however, mean the end of the patient's unconditional positive
regard for the therapist. The end of Herbert Marx's honeymoon, with the month's absence from treatment and the added
25 pounds, was marked by just such a shift in his feelings
towards me.

Freud saw in such reactions what he called a "negative
transference," the antithesis of the "positive transference"
which occurred when patients "transferred" their positive and
affectionate emotions onto the ostensibly neutral figure of the
psychoanalyst. Herbert's depreciation of me, as someone who
was "sincere" but "not qualified," suggested that his old
evaluation of his father as a weak and helpless person still
influenced his attitudes towards older men. Significantly, this
attitude towards me was evoked by circumstances in which
he felt helpless and abandoned to the overwhelming power
of his mother.

The most difficult aspect of Herbert Marx's negative
attitude was his breaking appointments. By simply absenting
himself from treatment, disappearing as his father had done
when he could no longer cope with the family environment,
Herbert could effectively stymie treatment in a way which
was peculiarly difficult to handle. If we couldn't talk about
what disturbed him, we could hardly resolve it. Long before
I began treating Herbert Marx, I had encountered this problem; and I had decided that no matter what the accepted
procedure was, I had to make vigorous efforts to encourage
the patient to continue treatment, as long as I felt that there
was any possibility of its successful outcome. It had therefore
become my practice to write patients, telephone them, and
take all kinds of measures to induce them to continue treatment.

At the time such activity on the part of a psychotherapist was generally viewed with disapproval. I remember Lewis Hill frowning upon evidences that a doctor might be getting too interested in the outcome of his patient's treatment. He repeatedly cautioned us against what he called "giving hostages," in the form of attention to patients which we might later fail to sustain out of accident or design. We were, for example, never to help a woman patient put on her coat unless we were prepared to continue this practice into the indefinite future.

Herbert Marx's attitudes towards me and towards the treatment were usually positive. Such attitudes had been prominent during the honeymoon phase of treatment, and they became more positive, in fact unrealistically so, during its latter phases. And they persisted even into his most depressed and despairing periods. On several occasions, when depression seemed to be impeding Herbert's ability to make progress in his treatment, it was possible to rely on these positive attitudes to get things moving again. For example, I would increase the frequency of our visits from once to twice and even three times a week. If the power of this relationship could extend over no more than the day of treatment, then at least there could be three such islands of tranquility in the course of his hectic week. From these islands, he could perhaps extend the feelings of refuge to more and more of the week.

Herbert shared this view. "Everything here is safe and free of anxiety. It's even more than that, it's like a shot of adrenalin. I always feel so good in here." Even during periods of profound discouragement he came to expect that he would feel better during our visits. "It's amazing how these sessions work. I've only been here ten minutes and I already feel that I could go out and do something, that the day is not completely ruined."

Once the increased frequency of visits seemed to have achieved its purpose, when Herbert's self-confidence had returned and treatment was moving again, we reduced the frequency of visits to once or twice a week. Usually he suggested the reduction and I welcomed his initiative. At such times he would have become involved in more activities and wanted the time and money which he was spending on treatment to invest in them. Such investment increased the importance of rewards outside the treatment, and decreased the gratification which he received from the treatment itself.

The purpose of this concern with the special therapeutic relationship, and with the healing element in psychotherapy, was not simply to make Herbert feel better. It was also to enlist his wholehearted participation in the therapeutic venture, and to evoke every possible idea that he could bring to bear upon his problems. Above all, I tried not to interfere in any way with the exercise of his creativity, for, in the last analysis, the success of treatment depended upon it. I would never, for example, have conceived of the strategy of writing to Gladys at a time when he desperately needed the relationship with her. That was his doing.

The special personal relationship, and the healing aspects of therapy, are important in their own right. But of greater importance is their contribution to the persuasion aspect of therapy, to the new learning which must occur if therapy is to be more than a happy experience and a pleasant memory. How does this understanding and this new learning come about?

As was mentioned earlier, the second process of psychotherapy is discerning the patient's problems and also his strengths. The process of discerning Herbert's problems began on the first day of treatment and continued until the last. Often it was unsuccessful, but the discipline of subjecting painful and obscure events to careful scrutiny gradually improved his powers of observation and made him better able to recognize the determinants of his behavior. At times his efforts resulted in greater understanding of painful and confusing events. At times we were able to bring order out of chaos.

The first time we worked out an understanding of a painful and confusing event was during the first period of depression at the end of the honeymoon. What was to become a dominant theme throughout treatment was first uncovered in connection with his giving up his job as waiter at his mother's insistence. The theme was "giving in to her and becoming her little boy." These discoveries first conveyed to Herbert something of the nature of the heretofore obscure forces which had swept through his life, bringing in their wake bleak helplessness and self-contempt.

There was a comparable experience during another period of binging and weight gain. It occurred at the time when Herbert's relationship with Gladys was becoming disturbingly ambiguous. With encouragement he was able to ask her about her feelings towards him. The answer was painful and it ushered in a second period of depression. But the episode was important, for it served as a model for forming and testing a hypothesis about a painful relationship. And it gave him some experience in dealing with such a relationship in a straightforward way.

Straightforward dealings with people had not been Herbert's strong suit. Nowhere was this more apparent than in his relationships with his mother; and over a period of time we examined some of his obscure and devious interactions with her. He learned to his surprise that this behavior had not been his own invention, but rather one he had learned from a skillful teacher.

One such episode stands out. It occurred during Herbert's first period of depression. He had declined an invitation to a Bar Mitzvah because he felt so inferior and believed that attending it would make him too uncomfortable. His mother knew the family which was holding the celebration and had heard about his declining the invitation. She wanted to find out the reason, but apparently could not bring herself to ask him directly. So she did it indirectly, by asking him if he would help her in the store on the day in question. He replied with some indignation, "How can I, Ma? You know I am going to the Bar Mitzvah."

There ensued a long sparring match, and eventually Herbert admitted having declined the invitation. Puzzled, I later pressed him for an explanation of this curious behavior.

There was an edge of anger in his voice as he said, "I did it because I wanted to make her squirm. I hate her deviousness."

The discernment of these various problems played an important part in Herbert's growing understanding. But the most important instance of growth during the first year of treatment required no special effort and occurred almost casually. Once the honeymoon phase of treatment had conferred a modicum of comfort, and he dared to hope, he decided, "I'm all set for the next step; now I want to have a date." And no longer setting the arbitrary weight barrier of reaching 160 pounds, he began to plan how to ask Gladys.

In helping him to screw up his courage, I found myself developing a treatment strategy which I have continued to use since then. The strategy consists, quite simply, of encouraging the patient to talk about a specific goal or aspiration. Once the patient begins to talk, I listen attentively, nodding encouragement, and indicating approval—anything to keep him talking about the goal. When he deviates from the topic, I look away, fail to respond, and give no encouragement.

Over the weeks I discovered that judicious application of attention could cause Herbert's talk about dating to move in ever more specific channels. First it was the rewards which he expected to gain from dating, then statements of confidence in his ability to overcome his fears, then more and more concrete plans, leading up to the idea of writing Gladys. And then finally came the day when he came into the office to announce that he had actually written to her. His exuberance was touching; and her prompt and friendly reply fully rewarded his initiative.

In encouraging Herbert to see Gladys these tactics seemed to work even more dramatically. Very small instances of attention were sufficient to keep him talking about dating her. And even when this conversation began with an account of his fears of meeting her, he would soon shift to more resolute statements and more hopeful fantasies. In less than a month his confidence about being able to see Gladys rose sharply, even though he had not yet seen her. I had only just begun to wonder whether he would continue to talk so bravely in the interviews and fail to act, when he told me that he had finally seen her. Again, the strategy seemed to have worked.

But the triumph was short-lived. When Gladys eventually rejected Herbert for another man, I discovered that my ability to modify the content of his talk almost disappeared. For whatever reason, and probably because my tactics were no longer rewarding to him in his depressed state, I found myself unable to interrupt the recurrence of his interminable ruminations about his eating, his body, and his despair.

Herbert's depression finally subsided, at the same time that he increased his ability to cope with his family. His interest in dating revived, and in these altered circumstances his responsiveness to my rewarding the content of his speech increased dramatically. So I immediately started reinforcing his talk about dating. Within a month he entered the office, radiating confidence, to announce, "I made a certain phone call today." His second experience in dating had begun.

This was the very same day on which he had left his uncle's house, telling his family he would look elsewhere for a place to live. In one fell swoop, Herbert tasted the fruits of success in both his social and his family relationships. It is difficult to say which was the more important in its favorable effect upon his body image. But whatever the cause, the effect was striking. Despite his weight of 240 pounds, Herbert was jubilant. "God knows why, but it's gotten so that I almost *feel* thin . . . I feel that I'm in command now." With these confident words, he entered a new phase of treatment; and we will continue his story from the previous chapter.

I soon had ample opportunity to examine the effects of this new strategy, for Herbert's second experience in dating turned out as unhappily as the first. But this time his reaction was far less intense. After a temporary halt, he returned to the quest with renewed enthusiasm. When one girl turned down his invitation, he simply called another. "I'm trying harder now than I ever did before. I know I'm going to get turned down and have unhappy experiences. But I'm going to keep trying until I get a date."

We reflected upon the difference from the year before, when his desperation had led to decreased activity and depression. Now it was leading to action. He no longer felt helpless. He was developing a sense of mastery about dating, and this was sufficient to make him feel optimistic. Systematically, he went about trying to get a date, with no special emotion and with low expectation of success. Over the weeks his effectiveness increased and his efforts paid off. Girls began to accept his invitations. But their acceptance was less important than it would have been formerly. "Just my asking them out is the important thing. It doesn't really matter so much whether I have a date or not as long as I can ask a girl for one."

This increased self-confidence spread into other areas of his life. "Today some nurses got in the elevator after I got on to come up to your office. This used to frighten me so much that I used to get out when they got in. I just felt that they would have complete disgust for me, total revulsion, because I was so fat. Today it didn't bother me at all. Now I'm thinking like a person of normal weight. I just think I'm doing the best I can. Not in respect to weight, of course, but in living the best way I can, not staying up too late at night, getting up in the morning on time, and when I study, studying the important things first and leaving the others till later, or even not doing them at all. No great fireworks, but it feels good."

Herbert found, when he began to date at the age of 23, that he really didn't know much about it. He had missed the typical experiences of his age group, and his naiveté resulted in some blunders. Once, for example, he decided to follow the advice of a classmate to "diversify"—to date different girls. But his diversification consisted of trying to date the best friend of a girl he was then dating.

But he continued to try and to learn from his efforts. And his experiences modulated the unrealistic fantasies he had dreamed during the years of loneliness. "I used to believe that people on dates are the most wonderful people in the world. Now I'm finding that they are just people after all, and dating is just like a lot of other things in life."

His increasingly realistic appraisal of dating and his determination to succeed at it made the process easier and easier. "It's almost like an adventure. I keep looking forward to seeing how things will turn out." Even disappointments could no longer set him back. For example, on one occasion he was turned down for a date by a girl he had come to like. "When I hung up the phone I felt crushed and terribly angry at her. I felt 'Goddamn women . . . who needs them anyway?' Then that evening I had a dream. I really can't remember the details. All I know is that I asked her to go out and she said yes." Herbert went on talking about the girl and his anger and how he felt: "I'll never ask you out again, sister. The hell with you. We're through." Then, as we talked further, he realized that he wanted very much to go out with her again and that his dream had been a simple fulfillment of this wish. He took a deep breath, sighed and smiled. Then he left the office and called her again.

Let me backtrack at this point to an earlier stage of Herbert's therapy in order to consider another aspect of treatment: helping the patient to discern his problems. Eating binges provided a good opportunity, for I had had considerable experience with them, and Herbert Marx had quite typical binges. He described their occurrence, as I had come to expect, as "sudden . . . unpredictable . . . out of the blue." He told of how they frightened him by showing the extent to which his life was controlled by irrational forces. I was able to tell him that my experience with other patients made me confident that his binges had quite specific causes. What is more, I told him, I believed that systematic, disciplined study of his binges would enable us to discover those causes. I told him that eventually I thought that he would be able to control the causes and, thus, the binges.

He took heart from this formulation and began paying attention to what preceded his binges. For a long time, his effort bore little fruit. During the honeymoon phase of treatment he had few binges. Then, when he became depressed, he felt too discouraged, particularly after a binge, to review in a disciplined manner what had preceded it. His efforts produced either detailed lists of minutiae or very general statements about feeling angry, bored, or frustrated.

Eventually, however, our low-keyed but insistent inquiry increased his awareness of events which preceded his binges. Nearly a year after treatment had begun, he said that he had been mulling over this matter and the anger which was usually present. "But there's something more than anger." He paused, frowned, and said slowly, "It's a feeling that someone is imposing their will on me."

Then Herbert had a binge which confirmed this supposition. It occurred during the period of exhiliration that had followed his first date with Gladys. A good part of this joy had stemmed from what he saw as Gladys's acceptance of him as a man—and one aspect of manhood, as he saw it, was the kind of clothes you wore. For years he had envied men who dressed in the Ivy League style which he had seen in the windows of men's stores. And for years he had let his uncle buy his clothes for him at the cut-rate, wholesale clothing store which belonged to a distant relative of the family.

Now, in the full flush of his newly-won manhood, he announced that he was going to buy himself an Ivy League suit at a men's store. The scene of this announcement was his aunt's house, and her righteous reaction stunned him: "Don't you go getting any ideas about buying clothes by yourself . . . And stay away from men's stores. If a men's store ever got its hands on a soft touch like you, they'd rob you blind."

He continued morosely, "It was just more of the same attitude that they've always had about me. I'm all right as a person who can memorize from books, but I don't know anything about the real world.

"Then my cousin said that if I really needed a new suit so badly she would go out and buy one for me. Then my aunt got into the act and said no, that my cousin wasn't going to buy any suit for me. There was no reason why my uncle shouldn't take me down to the wholesale dealer's like he'd always done, and that he knew good material when he saw it and wouldn't be cheated. It was like they were taking over . . . They seemed so positive."

For just a few moments Herbert had been angry, and then he began to back down. Their ideas seemed right. He began to wonder how he had ever thought that he would be able to buy a suit by himself. It somehow just seemed like the right thing for him to go down to the wholesale store with his uncle. "Then I noticed that I had this overwhelming desire to eat. So I left the house and went to a store around the corner and had myself an enormous binge."

As we continued to study Herbert's binges, we became able to distinguish their different elements. Frequently they were preceded by an interaction with someone who, as Herbert put it, "tried to impose his will on me." If he gave in, there was usually a period of tense anticipation. Thoughts of food would arise and become increasingly intense. Then came the binge, with all of its sequelae. Gradually we began to recognize that the critical time in this sequence was the period of discomfort between the precipitating circumstances and the actual eating. At first Herbert was quite unaware of any such period. Then, when he finally became aware of it, it was rarely more than four or five minutes before he found himself compelled to eat. As we continued to study individual binges, this interval increased, to an hour, or even two. When the interval became this long, we could begin to devise strategies for aborting the binge.

It seemed as if Herbert was experiencing intense, if sometimes poorly perceived, anxiety during this latent period. We therefore explored the possibility of his taking some medication during this critical time. With some misgivings, he began to carry in his pocket one or two tablets of a minor tranquilizer. When he thought that a binge was threatening, he was to take them. For some time this strategy didn't work at all. He could never be completely sure that a binge was actually impending, and he felt that it would be improper, even immoral, to take a tranquilizer unless he could be certain that he was about to have a binge. For a time only the onset of a binge could give him this certainty, and by then it was too late. Eventually, however, he became able to take the medication, even when he was in doubt about the imminence of a binge.

Not unexpectedly, this new attitude ushered in a period of fewer binges. We never knew for sure whether this favorable development was due to the pharmacological effects of the medication. Certainly the fact of doing something on his own behalf during critical situations made him feel less helpless and gave him a sense of mastery over situations which had formerly filled him with dread. From this time on he became increasingly able to use the occurrence of a binge to examine, and often to correct, what was going wrong in his life.

The next step was to help Herbert come to grips with his relationship with his mother. Hoping to increase his awareness of it, I resorted again to the technique of influencing the content of his talk. Whenever he told me of something his mother had said, I showed special interest and encouraged him to continue. Soon he was recounting the long, detailed, emotion-ridden descriptions of his dealings with his mother. As he became progressively caught up in these descriptions, he started asking his mother more and more about her feelings regarding obesity. In this active role, he became able to tolerate her vicious attacks upon obesity and obese people. The helpless, frightened boy who could deal with his mother only in devious and obscure ways gradually became an assured and careful investigator.

As Herbert continued to report ever more outrageous sentiments on the part of his mother, I detected a shift in his attitudes towards her. Initially he had seemed frightened as he described his mother's assaults; then he seemed awed. Soon I began to hear a note of incredulity, and, finally, anger. Carefully assessing the quality of his emotion, I made every effort to reward him for statements which showed evidences of assertiveness.

It was at this time that Herb received the note from his mother saying that he was a terrible disappointment to the people who loved him, and asking why he did not appreciate their love. This had aroused the first overt expression of anger towards her. He had slammed the letter upon my desk and snarled, "What the hell does she think she's doing, sending me letters like this?"

From this point on it was relatively easy to encourage similar statements and feelings. Soon afterwards, while describing how his aunts disparaged him, he made his intense vow, "I'll never allow them to do this to me again." And only two weeks later he took on his uncle, the first clear-cut expression of anger towards a family member that he could remember. Soon he found himself arguing, angrily and effectively, with his aunts.

It was several months before Herbert's new-found ability to struggle with members of his family extended to his mother. A typical interchange between the two helps illuminate this difficulty. It occurred regularly during the telephone calls which he made every evening at her request. She would begin the conversation with an account of her troubles and of how much she had suffered during the day. "After a while I get to feeling very sympathetic toward her. I get so that I want desperately to help her. I feel that I would do anything to help her because she is suffering so much. Then, just when I can hardly stand it any more, she tells me that it's all my fault because I am a pig and I eat so much. She keeps getting angrier and angrier as she talks about it and I get all mixed up. I feel that if my mother is angry, I'm so attached to her that I have to be angry too. But there is no one to be angry at except myself . . . By the time I hang up I'm feeling just terrible."

This kind of episode occurred so regularly and so consistently that I felt it must have deep roots. Herbert confirmed the speculation: "I remember once when I was little and Mother's Day was coming up. I knew how much Mother wanted to be loved, and I wanted to show her how much I loved her, so I went to my aunt and she helped me to get Mother a present. I wrapped it up for her and wrote a card telling her how much I loved her. Then Mother's Day came, and Mother wouldn't even accept the present. She said, 'No, no, I can't accept presents from my children because they don't love me.' "

As we continued to explore Herbert's relationship with his mother, we became aware of an entirely new element in his perception of her. He still saw her as a fierce, powerful person who could overwhelm him despite his best intentions. But now, side by side with this image, another began to appear, an image of a dangerously frail and vulnerable woman. It was an image which had been painted in large part by his aunts. From his earliest years he could remember them enjoining, "Don't get Mother upset!" He was never sure exactly why it was so important that Mother should not be upset, but he had a sense that there would be terrible repercussions.

"I thought maybe she would get sick, or that she would get so upset that she would insult the customers and we would lose the store and all our money. She's always talking about how sick she is. I'm afraid that if she gets upset this will make her even sicker." He paused and then went on, frowning, "I guess I really feel that if I make her angry it will kill her. I just can't take any chances on upsetting Mother." Again he paused. He shook his head as if incredulous over what he was about to say: ". . . *And if you upset Mother, you upset the balance of the world!*"

Discovering how vulnerable Herbert felt his mother to be took several months, and we spent several more discussing and clarifying his feelings about her. Gradually he relaxed the constraints against telling her how he felt. Two and a half years after he began treatment, he finally felt free enough to bring the quarrel into the open. The first round was a disaster.

He decided to do battle during the evening telephone call. He girded himself for her assault and prepared some choice remarks for replies. He waited until eleven o'clock at night in order to make sure she was alone. ". . . And when I reached her, she was still downstairs, working in the store. I just felt terrible about what I was planning to do. I really was ashamed of myself. I just couldn't go through with it."

If this evidence of his mother's back-breaking schedule aroused Herbert's guilt, she soon provided fuel for other feelings. ". . . I didn't call her yesterday so she called me. And she was just like a mad woman, hysterical and angry and striking out in all directions. She called me a pig. She said that I was so ugly and fat that of course girls didn't want to go out with me. She said that I might as well give up trying. She said she couldn't imagine a girl who would let me touch her."

Herbert went on. "Mother feels that my very being is loathsome." I agreed that this might be true, and reminded him that until a year or so ago he had felt the same way. Even now, occasionally, when he felt badly, these feelings would come back. We discussed why this should be so.

The viciousness of his mother's attacks could quite reasonably be interpreted as her unconditional rejection of him. But this interpretation frightened him. He had preferred to believe that her rejection was a conditional one, that he was being rejected, that is, because he was fat. This left some grounds for hope, for it implied that if he could only lose weight, then his mother would love him. "The thought that she might really hate me is just too terrible to imagine. So if she says that I'm a shit, I go out and prove that she's right by over-eating. My only hope is that the fault is in me and that I can change. If the fault is in her, then there's nothing to be done about it." Abruptly Herbert stopped. When he finally began again, it was with an expression almost of disbelief: "You know, all of a sudden I've gotten a terrible need to eat."

We continued another year. One by one we considered the obstacles to direct confrontation with his mother, and then resolved them. He later said that a major step in his emancipation from his mother was learning that she did not love him the way she said she did. When he had first heard of this notion, he said that it had been simply unbelievable. His aunts, and his mother herself, had told him so often how much she loved him that it had become an article of faith. After all, there were the incredible hours she worked in that miserable store simply to take care of him, put him through college, make him happy. "She was working so hard for me that I thought of her as a kind of god. I always felt that she was so loving that I didn't dare disagree with her about anything. I felt that I would be killing her if I disagreed."

Once Herbert was able to entertain the idea that his mother's love had its limits, things began to move. He grew to understand her harsh and humiliating comments for what they were. First he recognized her hostility; then he came to terms with it. Gradually he realized that he could not change his mother's view of him, even if he were to lose weight. Finally, he was able to cease the quest of winning her over, of making her happy by meeting her impossible terms. And he could go his own way.

Again and again in our interviews he rehearsed a new assertiveness towards his mother, speaking in angry terms of his plans to confront her. When the confrontation finally came, it was almost an anti-climax. After an active Sunday afternoon with friends, Herbert had stopped at the store for a brief visit. As was usual now, he was alert and prepared for trouble. Things went well until just before he left. Then, as he was walking out the door, his mother called after him, "Goodbye, stinker."

He raced back into the store ready for combat. Coldly he asked his mother what she meant by calling him "stinker." Then ensued a real-life version of the fantasied arguments he had enacted so often in my office and elsewhere. Even the presence of his aunt and a number of customers had not stopped him.

His mother met his unexpected outburst with a counterattack, demanding to know, "Do you love me or do you hate me?" Herbert replied that he had mixed feelings about her. To his delight his mother had replied, "No, you can't have mixed feelings. I'm the only one who can have mixed feelings." His mother went on to tell him of all that she had done for him and all that she had given him. He replied that he thought all of her gifts were simply ways of trying to enslave him. "I met every attack head on and I never lost my head. I won."

This battle with his mother marked the end of an era for Herbert Marx. From that point on, his activities took on a new ease and assurance. More and more he was master of his fate. Indeed, mastery became a prominent theme during his fifth, and last, year of treatment. It extended increasingly over his dieting, his dating, and his relations with his family, as well as his feelings about his work. He had always been a good student, but his work had never brought him the gratification it should have. Now, as he realized the fruits of his hard-won achievements in other areas, he came to appreciate his long-standing academic competence.

Herbert increasingly felt a sense of triumph. His growing mastery of his interpersonal problems had a profound effect upon both his disturbance in body image and his eating binges. The disturbance in body image essentially disappeared. The positive effects on his eating binges were not quite so potent. The binges became less frequent and less severe, but they never completely disappeared. Any one of a number of stresses, if he responded passively and with what he saw as self-betrayal, could precipitate an eating binge. It was usually a small one, however, and there was an encouraging aspect to it—its self-correcting nature. For the occurrence of even a small binge became a stimulus for Herbert to begin a careful analysis of the circumstances which had precipitated it; and the results of this analysis would move him towards more appropriate responses to the stress.

Once started, Herbert's competence in his relations with his family increased rapidly. He no longer permitted angry complaints about himself or his characteristics. He asserted himself earlier and earlier in the course of impending trouble. When he had gained some experience in the exercise of his anger in the family, he modulated it. It became easier and easier to achieve his ends by firm and decisive action; anger was less and less often necessary.

He even learned to cope with his mother without having to be angry. "Last time I was home, my cousin was there, and she asked if she could have the vacuum cleaner back, that she had loaned us. Mother told her that I would be glad to take the vacuum cleaner over to her house in my

car. It wasn't much, but I decided to do something about
it. I told Mother in a very stern voice to speak for herself,
and if she wanted me to do something for my cousin to ask
me first. One nice thing about it was that my uncle was there
and he heard everything. Later, when we were alone, he congratulated me."

Herbert's increased confidence finally manifested itself
in weight reduction. After all of the years of failure, this too
was almost an anticlimax. Three years after entering treatment
he embarked upon a reducing diet, quietly and with no dramatic show of determination. He continued on the diet without significant interruption, losing about ten pounds a month,
and reducing from 260 to his target weight of 140 pounds
in a year. Even more remarkable, his weight has not exceeded
145 pounds in the ten years and more since then.

His school work, which had always been good, now
became excellent. He completed his doctoral requirements
in the minimum time and obtained a promising job in industry. Dating was successful and easy. Once he acquired the
ability to date, he pursued it enthusiastically, as if to make
up for the lost years. For more than a year he "played the
field," dating a number of girls. Then one day, three and
a half years after he had entered treatment, Herb came into
the office and said that the last weekend had been the best
one he'd ever had. He had had two dates, but the one on
Saturday night had been special. "I liked her and she liked
me, and I guess that that's the first time that this has ever
happened. When I got back from the date, I told my roommate, 'I've met the girl I'm going to marry.' "

After all of the difficulties Herbert had had in accomplishing so much smaller ends, his courtship of Carol was
remarkably easy. They were married the following spring. He
continued to see me once a week during the first year of his
marriage, and I think that both of us were surprised at how
smoothly he adjusted to it. When problems did arise, they
were generally of a kind which we had dealt with many times
before, in far more aggravated form. His disciplined introspection could usually detect their origins and devise strategies

to cope with them with little help from me. It was heart-warming to watch the flowering of this fine young man after all of the painful years.

Soon after his engagement, Herbert happened to meet Jerome, his old college roommate. Jerome was lonely and unhappy, ". . . So Carol got a date for him and we're taking them skating with us this evening." He went on to explain, "I'm in love now, and when you're in love you feel so good that you want to help make other people feel good too."

On Valentine's Day, he told me proudly that he had sent valentines to every member of his family. It was the first time he had ever done this, the first time he had ever even had any inclination to do it. And it gave him a warm feeling as he thought about it. Remembering his unhappy Mother's Day years before, I shared that warmth.

During his first year of marriage, Herbert was given the opportunity of transferring to the West Coast branch of his company, with a major increase in pay and responsibility. Neither he nor Carol had ever lived outside Philadelphia, and for a time they discussed what it would mean to leave their families and friends. Then they decided to go out and look at the job. The visit was a successful one, and shortly after their return, they decided to move to the Coast.

Herbert told me about this decision and how, the evening that they made it, "I was wearing my Ivy League suit, and I went to the mirror in the bathroom and I looked at myself. Then I said, 'You're O.K., fellow. You may not be the smartest guy in the world, or the wittiest or the handsomest, but you're O.K.' "

He paused for a time, reminiscing, and then went on, "I thought about how different it used to be when I looked in the mirror, and how as soon as I looked, I would despise myself and say, 'You shit-head, you putz, you jerk.' I've come a long way since then . . ."

At our last meeting, Herbert spoke about the fight he had had with Carol's mother over their move. He had had a binge afterwards, but it hadn't discouraged him. We spent this last visit exploring the ways in which he had failed to assert himself with Carol's mother. He knew what he wanted to do; and he was sure that next time he would do it better.

Then our time was up. I had tears in my eyes when we said goodbye.

Since his move, I have seen Herbert only occasionally, and most of what I know about him is from letters which he sends me at Christmas. Three years after he left, he enclosed a snapshot "of our little pride and joy. She is a happy baby, but she is not nearly as happy as her parents are."

Last year he said simply, "We hope you are well. This has been a year of blessing for us: a new house, a new job (Chief of Section of my Division), and two children who make for hours of work and moments of sheer delight."

ten

Behavior Therapy

The treatment of Herbert Marx had been a long and profoundly moving experience for me. It also marked the end of my efforts to understand obesity through the long-term intensive study of individual patients.

He, and others like him, had taught me a decisive lesson. Psychotherapy could help obese people. Given enough time and effort it could relieve their disturbances in body image and help them control their eating binges. It could even help them lose weight and keep it off.

But this treatment had also taught me another lesson: we would have to look elsewhere to find economically justifiable means for controlling obesity. Individual psychotherapy is time-consuming and expensive. For too many patients, it is a hopelessly extravagant luxury.

But what are the alternatives? If individual therapy is impractical for the great mass of people suffering from obesity, where do we go from here? I have always believed that one day basic biochemical research will provide definitive means of managing obesity. But that could be a long way off, and what do we do until the biochemist arrives?

Happily, further progress has been made, beginning rather unexpectedly. One day on morning rounds, a resident in our Psychiatric Service gave a report on a patient with anorexia nervosa, the curious self-starvation of adolescent girls that was discussed earlier. It was an impressive presentation—warm, concerned, and human, with a scholarly review of the medical literature on the topic.

Anorexia nervosa is a very difficult condition to treat. Young women cling to their semi-starved way of life with incredible tenacity. This tenacity could be lessened by tranquilizers, and so we used them; and with large doses the patients usually began to eat more. But it was an uncertain course of treatment, frequently interrupted by obscure circumstances and sudden reversals. Behind it all lay the central irrationality of the illness—a fear of obesity so intense as to override the most powerful pangs of hunger, and ultimately even the hold on life itself.

The frustrations of trying to treat these women led the residents to search for anyone who might have any suggestions for helping. This search led them to John Paul Brady. An unusually able psychiatrist, he was a pioneer in the new and rapidly developing field of behavior therapy.

In general terms, behavior therapy consists of a variety of different therapeutic techniques, bound together by the belief that behavior disorders are learned responses, and that modern theories of learning have much to teach us about the acquisition and extinction of these responses.

Applying this framework to the treatment of anorexia nervosa, Brady helped the residents carry out a behavioral analysis of the problem. If, as Skinner claimed, behavior is maintained by its consequences, what were the consequences to these patients of eating and of refusing to eat? Most of them acknowledged that eating, even the prospect of eating, was consistently frightening. Some were more explicit. They told of their fear that any food intake whatsoever would lead to a total breakdown of their resolve and to an orgy of eating binges. Their refusal to eat relieved that anxiety.

Taking this a step further, Brady suggested the following: if the refusal to eat was maintained by the relief of anxiety, it could perhaps be overcome by following eating with some reward that was more powerful than the anxiety which was its usual consequence. But what reward could possibly compete with the pervasive anxiety with which these girls had learned to live?

The search for rewards did not at first look promising. One of the striking characteristics of patients with anorexia nervosa is a widespread inhibition against most normal activity. Tense and frozen in appearance, they are a cheerless lot, for whom all pleasure and satisfaction seem to have long-since departed. It was hard on the face of it to think of anything they might find rewarding. Then a related study suggested a possible approach.

We had been using pedometers to investigate the physical activity of anorexia patients, looking into the as yet unsubstantiated belief that they are unusually active. The results began to come in, just when we needed them, clearly demonstrating that physical activity was indeed very important to these patients. Was it important enough to start them eating again? Brady proposed that the residents find out by making the opportunity for physical activity dependent upon eating (or, its consequence, weight gain). Specifically, he proposed that each anorexia patient be given a six-hour pass to leave the hospital on any day that her morning weight was at least half a pound above her previous morning's weight. No further intervention of any kind was to be made. The residents were to make no comment about the patients' level of activity, food consumption, or body weight. The program was simply to be explained to them and then carried out.

The first resident to tell his patient about the new rules was met with an explosion of fury, and threats to run away from the hospital. The nurses were subjected to equally angry outbursts, and then pitiful pleading that she be let out of the building for walks, whether or not she gained weight.

Four days after the new program was instituted, this patient's morning weigh-in showed a weight gain of nearly a pound. She stopped complaining, and during the next week gained almost six pounds. This surprising change continued, with weight gains of five pounds a week. And that wasn't all. Her tense, frozen manner thawed; she began to seek out and talk with other patients and nurses. She reported that she felt better, and her voice and manner made it clear that she did.

These results made a very strong impression on me. For years I had known about the difficulties of treating people with anorexia nervosa, and although I had personally treated only a few, I had learned to be satisfied with limited goals and long hospitalizations. Suddenly, here was a disarmingly simple technique, proposed by someone with no special expertise in dealing with this illness. What really made me sit up and take notice was that it worked. Inevitably, I began to think about its application to the treatment of obesity. If such a simple program could be so effective in a condition as stubborn as anorexia nervosa, why couldn't a similar approach help obese people to lose weight?

During the next several months I applied these ideas to the treatment of a small number of intelligent, well-motivated obese people. Each day that they lost weight they would be rewarded by some highly-prized activity and freedom from some chores, in an effort to establish the kind of contingency which had been so successful with the anorexics. In each instance the result was the same: after an initial weight loss of 10 or 15 pounds, the patient had stopped losing weight. The technique wasn't entirely without effect. Careful study of the weight patterns revealed that the program did seem to have some influence, but it was disappointingly weak and short-lived.

Reluctantly, I drew the conclusion that behavior therapy was not useful in the treatment of obesity. Despite the promise held out by the experience with anorexia nervosa, my efforts had not had any more effect than the myriad of other treatments which had come and gone over the years.

I felt quite confident about this decision, since my earlier review of the medical literature on obesity had revealed a striking consistency in the results of outpatient treatment.[18] No matter what treatment was used, no more than 25 percent of the patients lost as much as 20 pounds, and only 5 percent lost as much as 40 pounds. Unless a treatment program could improve on these results, there was no reason to believe that it had any special merit. And I wasn't even doing this well.

Just when I had finally decided that behavior therapy could not help obese people, Paul Brady sent me a copy of a short article in a little-read behavior therapy journal. I could hardly believe my eyes when I read it. For in this report on "Behavioral Control of Overeating,"[19] Richard Stuart, then a Professor of Social Work at the University of Michigan, reported the best results that had ever been obtained in the outpatient treatment of obesity. The paper remains a landmark in the field.

The graphs of weight loss of eight patients over a one-year period showed a steady steep downward course. Not 25 percent, but *all* eight patients had lost more than 20 pounds. Not 5 percent, but *50 percent* had lost more than 40 pounds.

Sitting there in the office looking over the paper I had a profound sense of its significance. Stuart's work was the first major advance in the treatment of obesity in 30 years. And oddly enough, he had no idea of the excitement that was to be ignited by his research.

He had chosen obesity as a subject of study for two simple reasons: it provided a convenient and objective measure of the effectiveness of the treatment (i.e. pounds lost); and a detailed description of a behavioral program for obesity was already available, from an early study by Charles Ferster.[20] Stuart had had no thought of breaking any records. And because at that time he didn't know a great deal about obesity, he did not at first realize how remarkable his results really were.

Ferster's program had produced negligible weight losses; Stuart's were dramatic. What had he done that made the difference? I returned to the reports to find the answer, but it wasn't apparent. There were a few small differences, but they could hardly account for the large variation in outcomes.

Stuart had treated his patients individually; Ferster had carried out his treatment in groups. Surprisingly, Stuart had actually seen his patients fewer times; instead of Ferster's regular weekly meetings, he had concentrated his efforts at the beginning of the treatment. He saw patients for 30-minute sessions 3 times a week for the first 12 to 15 sessions. During the next three months, he scheduled treatment sessions as needed, usually at two-week intervals. Thereafter he saw patients monthly, and then finally, for "maintenance" sessions as needed. The total number of sessions during the year varied from 16 to 41.

Except for these differences in form and frequency, the methods used by the two investigators were quite similar, and Stuart gave full credit to Ferster's early work. One of the virtues of this work had been its meticulously detailed description of methods. This explicitness (which has been a perennial goal of behavior therapists) made these programs applicable to far more than Stuart's eight original patients. The clearly described "how to do it" instructions allowed others to learn exactly what Ferster and Stuart had done. So we set about seeing if we could do it too.

Much of the work was carried out by Sydnor "Pete" Penick, a remarkably productive young physician, who was already an experienced obesity researcher. Acting on his initiative, we decided to go a step beyond Stuart and compare patients treated by behavior therapy with others treated by conventional methods. It seemed wildly improbable, but who could say—perhaps this unknown Richard Stuart was a therapeutic genius who would have done as well with any method. Only the use of a control group could tell us for sure that it was the behavior therapy and not some special virtue of the therapist which had made the difference.

But what kind of control group should we use? Pete proposed that we put behavior therapy to the acid test: compare it with the most effective possible alternative. And what was that? Why clearly it was his own treatment, a composite of every method he knew of, except those described by Stuart. He included as a co-therapist a research nurse with extensive experience in the treatment of obesity. For the behavior therapy, we also selected a man and woman team, and again loaded the dice against behavior therapy by choosing therapists who had had no previous experience in behavior therapy. For that matter, they had had very little experience in treatment of any kind.

This contrast in therapists provided a critical test of behavior therapy. If the behavior therapy patients lost more weight than those in traditional treatment, despite the inexperience of their therapists, it would seem that it had to be behavior therapy which made the difference.

For weeks the inexperienced therapists worked over Ferster's and Stuart's papers, selecting out anything that looked like it might work. Even after the beginning of therapy, they continued to develop their program, using their growing understanding of behavior therapy and of the individual patients to try out new techniques and omit others which were not working.

This strategy of putting everything but the kitchen sink into the treatment program was a wise one. The first question we wanted to answer was: does behavior therapy work? Can it produce greater weight loss than more traditional means? If it couldn't, it would have been pointless to search out the effective elements of the treatment. If, on the other hand, the bulging package of behavior therapy techniques *did* produce greater weight loss than more conventional ones, we would know that at least some of these techniques had been effective. And there would then be plenty of time to dissect out the more effective ones. All too many carefully crafted

studies have wasted time and money because of the failure
to observe this simple principle: if you can't demonstrate the
effectiveness of a treatment, there isn't much purpose in elucidating its fine points. Or, if a study isn't worth doing, it isn't
worth doing well.

The patients who were treated in this carefully planned
program were more or less typical of those overweight people
who fill a large part of the practice of family physicians.
Generally in good health, middle-aged, middle class and predominantly women, they averaged 80 percent over their ideal
weight.

Fifteen patients were chosen at random to receive behavior therapy; an equal number received the best "traditional"
treatment that Pete Penick could devise. Over a three month
period, each group (averaging seven or eight) met weekly for
two hours.

The behavioral program had four parts to it: (1) a description of the behavior to be controlled (eating), (2) control
of the stimuli that precede eating, (3) techniques to control
the act of eating, (4) prompt reinforcement of behaviors that
delay or control eating.

Description of the behavior to be controlled. The patients
were asked to keep careful records of the food they ate. Each
time they ate they wrote down precisely what it was they
had eaten, how much was eaten, the time of day, where they
were, and how they felt. The immediate reaction of most
patients to this time-consuming and inconvenient procedure
was grumbling and complaints. In retrospect, this negative
response may well have been due to our own initial uncertainty
about the technique. Since then, as we have become convinced
of its effectiveness, and have wholeheartedly stressed its importance, patients have responded more positively. In fact, most
patients have come to share our view that record-keeping may
be the single most important part of the program. It vastly
increases their awareness of how much they eat, of the speed
with which they eat, and the large variety of environmental
and psychological situations associated with eating. Despite

their years of struggle with the problem, most patients express surprise when they learn from the record-keeping how much they eat and the circumstances surrounding their eating.

Sometimes the record-keeping alone produced surprising results. A middle-aged traveling salesman came to realize for the first time that he over-ate only in his car, which he kept liberally stocked with candy bars, peanuts and potato chips. He thought over the problem, stopped storing food in the car, and promptly lost weight.

Record-keeping helped another patient, a 30-year-old housewife, make a similar discovery: for the first time in her life she realized that anger caused her to over-eat. Having made this discovery she acted upon it. Whenever she found herself getting angry, she would make every effort to leave the kitchen or any place where food was available, and if there were time, she would write down how she felt. She became increasingly able to avoid eating in response to anger, and began to lose weight.

A few weeks of simple record-keeping was sometimes more effective in making people aware of their eating patterns than even long-term intensive psychotherapy. This contrast was particularly dramatic in the case of a Philadelphia matron who had been quite satisfied with her five years of psycho-therapy, judged by her psychiatrist to be fairly successful.

"Even though I started psychotherapy because of my weight, as far as the psychotherapy was concerned I don't think it proved anything about weight. It just didn't have anything to do with weight reduction. It made me infinitely more content with myself. It helped me to live with myself the way I am. But it didn't have any lasting effect on how I ate.

"The strongest part of the behavior therapy program was the realization of what you were eating. My problem—and I think it's shared by a lot of people—was that I really had no conception at all of what I ate. When I was in the kitchen, I would just go from one place to the other and pick up things and eat them, without any idea of what I ate or even that I had eaten at all. Keeping those records made me recognize what I was eating, but writing it down became one terrible bloody bore. I felt I just had to do it, and so I did, but I never liked it."

Control of the stimuli that precede eating. The stimuli which precede eating, and particularly the so-called "discriminative stimuli," play a large part in the eating which follows them. The concept of a discriminative stimulus comes from the animal laboratory, where such stimuli as the flashing of a light or the sounding of a tone may be a signal to an animal that pressing a lever will produce food pellets or other rewards. Since the reward never occurs without the discriminative stimulus, the stimulus is said to "control" the behavior which is rewarded.

The patients' records showed that their eating occurred in a wide variety of places and at many different times during the day. Some noted that if they ate while watching television, for example, it was not long before watching television made them eat. It was as though the various times and places had become discriminative stimuli controlling eating.

In an effort to decrease the number and potency of the stimuli which controlled their eating, patients were encouraged to confine eating, including snacking, to one place. So as not to disrupt domestic routines, this place was usually the kitchen.

A parallel effort was made to develop new discriminative stimuli for eating, and to increase their power. Patients were encouraged, for example, to use distinctive table settings, perhaps a uniquely colored place mat and napkin, with special silver. We made no effort to reduce the amount of food the patients ate, but we did urge them to use the distinctive table setting whenever they ate, even when it was only a between-meals snack.

Several patients carried out these suggestions with great conscientiousness. One diligent housewife, convinced of the importance of this measure, went so far as to take her table setting with her whenever she dined out. She lost weight early and easily. Was it because she had controlled her discriminative stimuli for eating? Perhaps it was; we don't yet know for sure.

Once patients were able to stop pairing their eating with such activities as reading the newspaper and watching television, we encouraged them to make further efforts to make eating a pure experience. They were urged to do whatever they could to make meals a time of comfort and relaxation, and particularly to avoid old arguments and new problems at the dinner table. They were encouraged to savor the food they ate, to make a conscious effort to become aware of it as they were chewing, and to enjoy the act of swallowing and the warmth and fullness in their stomachs.

Development of techniques to control the act of eating.   One of the major difficulties in controlling the size of a meal is the fact, discussed in relation to the glucostatic theory, that no more than a small fraction of the meal is absorbed until at least 20 minutes after it has begun. Solely from the point of view of physical satiation, there is consequently much to recommend a slowing in the rate of eating. Furthermore, such slowing heightens awareness of all the components of the eating process and makes it easier to gain control over them. For these reasons we developed specific techniques to help the patients eat more slowly.

They were urged to count each mouthful of food, or each chew, or each swallow. They were encouraged to practice putting down their eating utensils after every third mouthful, until it had been fully chewed and swallowed. Then longer delays were introduced, starting with one minute towards the end of the meal when it was more easily tolerated, and moving to longer and more frequent delays, and then to ones earlier in the meal.

These techniques and those designed to control the discriminative stimuli produced some enthusiastic testimonials. Among the more enthusiastic were those of Mary O'Brien, a college student whose poise and skillful dressing artfully obscured her 180 pounds. She reported her excitement at the first meeting after Thanksgiving.

"It's the very first time in my life that I can remember getting through Thanksgiving without over-eating, and it was the things we learned here that helped me. I just concentrated on eating slowly, and the first thing I knew the dinner was over and I hadn't had seconds. I even left some of the food on the plate!" She continued this practice, and continued to surprise herself. "A couple of nights ago when I was studying I went into my roommate's room and took a cookie, just *one cookie*, from a box that she had there. I ate it very slowly, chewing it carefully and tasting every part of it. And then I went back to my room to study. I was in absolute awe of myself—was this the same Mary O'Brien who two months ago wouldn't have been able to stop at *ten cookies*, let alone one?—who would have eaten the whole box and then another one if it was there?"

William Schultz, a huge, burly man with a full beard and a hearty laugh, entered the program proclaiming he was a "pessimist." "I've lost weight before—I even lost 80 pounds once—and I've always regained it. I suppose I'll lose weight in this program, but I don't have any confidence at all that I will be able to keep it off."

A month later, shaking his head in disbelief, he reported, "You know, it's amazing. I don't know what's done it. I don't know whether it was slowing down, or concentrating and making it a pure experience or what . . . But when I did these things I really tasted food for the very first time in my life. I *really tasted food!* I can't get over it. When somebody used to ask me if I liked food, I would always say 'Sure I like it.' But I'd never really tasted it before. Before, I could eat half a gallon of ice cream at one sitting and never really taste a single bit of it. Now I eat one spoonful of ice cream and really taste it, and it gives me as much pleasure as a whole half gallon used to."

Prompt reinforcement of behaviors which delay or control eating. Although we, as Ferster and Stuart before us, devised elaborate systems of reinforcement, I think that the most effective rewards were informal ones, incidental to the structured aspects of the program. Perhaps the most important of these was the great sense of satisfaction which patients developed with their growing exercise of control over eating.

With Herbert Marx still very much on my mind, I remembered how long it had been before patients in more traditional therapy began to talk about feelings of control, and of how important these feelings had been to them. As a result, I was surprised and delighted with the speed with which these feelings began to appear in behavior therapy. In many ways this effect was like the equally unexpected influence of the behavioral program on the anorexia nervosa patients—when their weight gain was matched by a relief from tension and by the development of warmth in their social relations.

As Mary O'Brien explained, "It's like I'm making my own future. I think that what it comes down to is that I've started to take control of my life; it's in my hands now to shape and mold as I see fit. It started with controlling my eating, but now it's much more than my eating. Maybe that's because eating has always meant so much to me."

Mr. Schultz, no longer a pessimist, reported that his wife had asked him if he had increased the number of tranquilizers he was taking because he seemed so calm. "She just couldn't get it through her head that I not only hadn't increased the tranquilizers, I had stopped taking them altogether. I don't know quite why I feel so good, but probably it's because I feel that I'm calling the shots now. I'm in control. But I sure as hell don't understand it. It's too easy—it ought to hurt."

One of the major problems of any behavioral program is how to reward the patient promptly after desired behavior. Every obese person has had some experience with rewards, but usually they have been too infrequent and too long delayed. As one housewife put it, "Like my husband might offer to buy me a car if I lost 50 pounds. And I might knock myself out and lose 30 pounds, which is a lot of weight. But what did it get me—half a car? I got nothing."

To be effective a reward must be administered promptly following performance of the behavior it is to modify. Even

a delay until the next weekly meeting is too long. In order
to decrease the interval between the behavior and its reward,
we devised a system which awarded the patient a certain
number of points immediately after each of the activities we
were trying to encourage: record-keeping, counting bites and
swallows, pausing during the meal, eating in one place, and
so on. These effectively provided immediate reward, and as
we gained experience, we added increasingly sophisticated
schedules, such as doubling the number of points earned when
a patient devised and performed an activity which was an
alternative to eating, in the face of strong temptation.

Arrangements with the patients' spouses permitted them
to convert their points into personal rewards: relief from house-
keeping chores, trips to the movies, and money, which they
brought to the next meeting for a donation to the group.
At the beginning of the program the patients decided how
the money should be used. To our surprise they chose very
altruistic courses. Each week the first group donated its savings
to the Salvation Army; the second gave its earnings to a needy
friend of one of the members.

We also devised a system to reward patients for weight
loss, in addition to behavior change. Here we tried to steer
a course between small weight losses which were not a result
of dieting, and weight losses so large that any rewards would
be dishearteningly distant. Patients and their spouses worked
out many of these rewards. Some were conventional, like a
trip to the movies for each five pounds lost, or a new dress
for 10 pounds. Others were highly creative. One which became
very popular required each patient to buy a pound of suet,
cut it into 16 pieces and place them in a plastic bag in a
prominent place in the refrigerator. The patient then attempted to visualize this as fat on her body. Every time she
lost a pound, she removed one ounce of fat from the bag
and tried to imagine its disappearance from her body. If she
gained weight, she added an ounce of fat to the bag for each
pound gained. When the bag was entirely empty, the group
gave her, along with lavish praise, a small prize such as a
book or a box of cosmetics.

What were the results of this program? As I mentioned earlier, the proportion of obese patients in the medical literature who lost 20 or more pounds was 25 percent; for losses of 40 or more pounds it was 5 percent. In our control group, treated by conventional methods, the results were very similar: 24 and 0. By contrast, the percent of patients treated by behavior therapy was 53 and 13! The difference was even more striking when judged on the basis of a weight loss of 30 pounds. None of the control patients lost this much; 33 percent of the behavior therapy patients did.

There were two other noteworthy effects of the program. None of the patients dropped out of treatment, in contrast to the strikingly high drop-out rates (from 20 to 80 percent) with conventional treatment. And none of the patients reported ill effects of any kind from the program.

In judging the effectiveness of behavior therapy, these were pertinent considerations. There was another of at least equal importance: how long was the weight loss maintained? It is generally believed that weight lost with reducing diets is rapidly regained; and the few scattered studies on the topic support this viewpoint. But the sad truth is that so few patients have lost any significant amount that the question of maintenance of weight loss has been largely irrelevant. If, however, behavior therapy were to prove a more effective method than those previously available, the question of maintenance would become considerably more relevant. With this in mind, we contacted each of the patients a year after treatment.

The results were surprisingly good. Each of the eight patients who had lost more than 20 pounds had maintained that weight loss; and three of them had lost an additional 20 pounds. Furthermore, one of the patients who had lost 40 pounds during treatment had by this time achieved a weight loss of over 100 pounds.

There was one more intriguing finding. Whereas the patients treated by traditional methods all lost about the same amount of weight, there was great variability in the weight losses of the behavior therapy patients. The five best performers belonged to this group as did the single least effective one, the only patient who actually gained weight during treatment. What does greater variability mean?

No one knows for sure, but the possibilities are intriguing. The weight loss of patients treated by traditional means, which was lower and more constant, suggests the effect of some non-specific factor that is common to all treatment—perhaps the establishment of a therapeutic relationship and the hope which it may evoke. The greater weight loss and its greater variability in the behavior therapy patients suggests that it may be brought about by a more specific factor, one which is particularly effective for certain patients and of little or no help to others. The greater variability thus may imply a greater specificity of behavior therapy.

It has another important implication. If we could predict ahead of time which patients were likely to respond to behavior therapy and which were not, we could concentrate our efforts on the former and increase their chances of success. At the same time we could save the latter patients from one more experience with failure. Unfortunately our attempts at prediction were unsuccessful, as have been those of others before and after us. Our experience with one patient offers a clear example of the difficulty in predicting outcomes.

Joseph Romolo was a 420-pound man in his late twenties, who was referred by the Department of Welfare. He had no job skills, had never held a steady job and had not had any job for years. After a slow start, he learned not only the techniques of behavior therapy but also the ideas which underlay them. (He devised a similar program to help himself stop smoking and followed it successfully.) Much to our surprise, he was one of the two patients who lost more than 40 pounds in the course of treatment. In fact, he was the one who subsequently went on to lose more than 100 pounds. When we last heard from him, he had completed a vocational rehabilitation course and had been at work for over a year. Yet even with the power of hindsight, I don't know now how we could have predicted his success.

This lack of predictability aside, the results of our first trial of behavior therapy were impressive—and not just in terms of weight lost. Even more striking was the increased self-esteem and well-being of those who mastered the technique. But we had to ask, as we had so often before with new treatments for obesity, was this just another fad? To what extent were the effects due merely to the support of the group and our own enthusiasm? How much resulted from the evocation of hope, hope which had so often before led obese people to lose weight and then been followed by disappointment?

The answer was not long in coming. Many research workers have been drawn to this field. The clear description of treatment methods and of the principles underlying them have made it feasible to reproduce treatments with a precision never before possible in research on psychotherapy. Research workers are also attracted by the precision and economy of weight loss as a measure of change. In comparison with the elaborate rating scales necessary to measure changes in anxiety and depression, and the crudeness and unreliability of the results, weight change in pounds is an investigator's dream. Not surprisingly, the past eight years have seen an explosion of research on the behavior therapy of obesity.

In study after study, behavior modification has been systematically compared with a wide variety of alternate treatment methods. And in every instance, those people treated with behavior modification have lost more weight. This kind of unanimity is unprecedented in psychotherapy research.

Given this effectiveness, are there ways that this treatment can be brought to bear upon larger populations? The answer is an emphatic "yes."

The great American love affair with weight reduction has already shown us one way—the patient-self-help group. A century and half ago De Tocqueville described the tendency of Americans to organize informal groups to achieve the ends that are the function of government in other societies. Nowhere is this proclivity more impressively expressed than in the organization of people to cope with a common illness.

One of the largest and most effective of these organizations is TOPS (Take Off Pounds Sensibly), with an enrollment of 350,000 members in 15,000 chapters across the country. It looked as if TOPS might be an ideal vehicle for a broad-scale introduction of behavioral techniques for the control of obesity. So we approached them and enlisted their cooperation in a study of the feasibility of introducing behavioral techniques on a grand scale.

Our study of 234 obese people in 16 TOPS chapters demonstrated the enormous potential of this organization.[21] Behavior modification could be introduced with surprising ease into TOPS, either by a psychiatrist, or, of even greater importance, by a TOPS chapter leader who was provided with the manual used by the psychiatrists and brief instruction in its use. Furthermore, the eight chapters treated by behavior modification lost significantly more weight than the four chapters which received a program of nutrition education, or the four chapters which continued the usual TOPS program. And the chapters which were treated by TOPS leaders lost almost as much weight as those treated by the psychiatrists.

The implications of these results are far-reaching. For if this new and more effective treatment had access to the multiplier effect of an organization of 350,000 people, the potential would be unprecedented. For the first time it would make possible a program large enough to affect the health of the nation.

The issue is still in doubt, but the signs are not favorable. For TOPS has made no effort to capitalize on the program which it helped to pioneer. Ironically, the chief beneficiaries may well be TOPS' arch rivals, the profit-making organizations. To date, there has been only limited investigation of these commercial weight reduction enterprises. But research is now under way; and within a short time we should know a great deal more about the effectiveness of this rapidly growing area. What we already know suggests that such approaches to health care may provide an attractive middle ground between the often unavailable and frequently over-specialized care by the individual physician on the one hand, and the broad social changes which can favorably alter life styles on the other.

The performance of the most prominent of the commercial organizations, Weight Watchers, suggests that private industry may well be the most potent agent for the widespread control of obesity in this country. The appeal of Weight Watchers, for example, far outstrips that of either medical auspices or self-help groups. In its 13 years of operation its membership has grown to two and a half million—seven times that of TOPS. Furthermore, Weight Watchers has shown great initiative in developing behavioral techniques for its programs, having recruited for this purpose the same Richard Stuart who ignited the explosion of behavioral research in obesity eight years ago.

It seems likely that other profit-making organizations will challenge Weight Watcher's virtual monopoly of the commercial weight reduction field and the field will develop rapidly. The next few years may well see a significant increase in the ability to control the critical social influences which affect obese people, as the genius of private industry enlists them in large-scale programs of behavioral control. If this development is coupled, as it probably will be, with further increase in the effectiveness of behavioral methods, we may well witness a phenomenon unprecedented in the history of medicine: management of a major health problem passing out of medical hands and into those of private industry.

These developments are particularly important in light of the major health problems of our time. With the conquest of infectious disease, these remaining problems are largely chronic ones, indissolubly linked to our life styles. Our leading killer, heart disease, which presently accounts for over half of all deaths in America, is a case in point. Except for heredity, every factor known to contribute to heart disease is a matter of personal habit: eating foods high in cholesterol and saturated fatty acids, smoking, inadequate physical activity, insufficient attention to the control of diabetes and high blood pressure, and . . . obesity.

All this can be changed by programs already underway. It is perhaps fitting to end this account on the threshold of these important new developments. I began this research with an attempt to discover something about obesity. Over twenty years later, the exploration continues. We have moved from explanation to action, as we are adding to the old questions of *why* people are obese, new questions of *how* to control obesity. It now appears that a broad scale assault on obesity need not await further biochemical knowledge.

Understanding its social determinants may be enough. The many-sided research on modifying these determinants, already fruitful, gives every promise of continuing productivity.

The problems of obesity are still far from solved. Even the application of our best available technology leaves huge numbers of obese people unhappy and in ill health. But for the first time in many years research already underway gives promise of aid and comfort in the foreseeable future. And this is just the beginning.

References

1. (p. 15) Fromm-Reichmann, F. Contribution of the Psychogenesis of Migraine. *The Psychoanalytic Review,* 24: 26–33, 1937.
2. (p. 36) Stunkard, A.J., Van Itallie, T.B., and Reiss, B.B. The Mechanism of Satiety: Effect of Glucagon on Gastric Hunger Contractions in Man. *Proceedings of the Society of Experimental Biology and Medicine,* 89: 258–261, 1955.
3. (p. 36) Seed, J., Acton, F. and Stunkard, A.J. A Model for the Appraisal of Glucose Metabolism. *Clinical Pharmacology and Therapeutics,* 3:191–215, 1962.
4. (p. 37) The Regulation of Hunger and Appetite. *Annals of the New York Academy of Sciences* (R.W. Miner, ed.), 63:1–144, 1955.
5. (p. 37) Body Composition. *Annals of the New York Academy of Sciences* (J. Brozek, ed.), 110:1–1018, 1963.
6. (p. 37) *Annual Review of Physiology* (J. Comroe, ed.). 33:533–568, 1971.
7. (p. 63) Stunkard, A.J., Grace, W.J. and Wolff, H.G. The Night-Eating Syndrome. A Pattern of Food Intake among Certain Obese Persons. *American Journal of Medicine,* 19:78–86, 1955.
8. (pp. 84, 86) Stunkard, A.J. The Dieting Depression: Incidence and Clinical Characteristics of Untoward Responses to Weight Reduction Regimens. *The American Journal of Medicine,* 23:77–86, 1957.
9. (p. 88) Stunkard, A.J. and Rush, A.J. Dieting and Depression Reexamined: A Critical Review of Reports of Untoward Re-

sponses During Weight Reduction for Obesity. *Annals of Internal Medicine,* 81:526–533, 1974.

10. (p. 141) Leary, T. *The Interpersonal Diagnosis of Personality.* Ronald Press, New York, 1957.

11. (p. 143) Srole, L., Langner, T.S., Michael S.T., et al. *Mental Health in the Metropolis: The Midtown Manhatten Study.* McGraw-Hill, New York, 1962.

12. (p. 151) Goldblatt, P.B., Moore, M.E. and Stunkard, A.J. Social Factors in Obesity. *Journal of the American Medical Association,* 192:1039–1042, 1965.

13. (p. 154) Mullins, A.G. The Prognosis in Juvenile Obesity. *Archives of Diseases of Children,* 33:307–313, 1958.

14. (p. 179) Stunkard, A.J. and Mendleson, M. Obesity and the Body Image: I. Characteristics of Disturbances in the Body Image of Some Obese Persons. *American Journal of Psychiatry,* 123:1296–1300, 1967.

15. (p. 182) Stunkard, A.J. and Burt, V. Obesity and the Body Image: II. Age at Onset of Disturbances in the Body Image. *American Journal of Psychiatry,* 123:1443–1447, 1967.

16. (p. 183) Hirsch, J. and Knittle, J.L. Cellularity of Obese and Nonobese Human Adipose Tissue. *Federation Proceedings,* 29:1516–1521, 1971.

17. (p. 191) Frank, J.D. *Persuasion and Healing.* Johns Hopkins University Press, Baltimore, 1961.

18. (p. 217) Stunkard, A.J. and McLaren-Hume, M. The Results of Treatment of Obesity: A Review of the Literature and Report of a Series. *Archives of Internal Medicine,* 103:79–85, 1959.

19. (p. 217) Stuart, R.B. Behavioral Control of Overeating. *Behavior Research and Therapy,* 5:357–365, 1967.

20. (p. 217) Ferster, C.B., Nurnberger, J.I. and Levitt, E.B. The Control of Eating. *Journal of Mathematics,* 1:87–109, 1962.

21. (p. 230) Levitz, L.S. and Stunkard, A.J. A Therapeutic Coalition for Obesity: Behavior Modification and Patient Self-help. *American Journal of Psychiatry,* 131:423–427, 1974.

Two books not referred to in the text are of particular value to anyone interested in a more systematic presentation of the subject of obesity. They are:

Mayer, J. *Obesity: Causes, Cost and Control.* Prentice-Hall, Englewood Cliffs, N.J., 1968.

Bruch, H. *Eating Disorders: Obesity, Anorexia Nervosa and the Person Within.* Basic Books, New York, 1973.

Index